MW01003953

Broken Hallelujah

40 Days in the Wilderness

A true story from:

MK and Matt Podschweit

Co-Authored by: Brenda Schaefer

ISBN: 9781790315741

ISBN-13:

For the Hospital Staff

That never gave up

For our families

Who never stopped believing

For our two girls

Aubrey Kathryn and Emily Grace

Love Wins, Always

For our dear friend

Brenda Schaefer

Thank you

Chapters

Preface

Broken Hallelujah was written for the following people:

— Black, White, Brown

— Jews, Hindus, Christians, Islamic, Atheists

— Redheads, Blondes, Brunettes, Bald

— Left-Handers, Right-Handers, Ambidextrous

— Male, Female

— Straight, Bisexual, Lesbian, Homosexual, Transgender

— Victims of Sexual Assault, Victims of Rape

— Addicted, Bullies, Bullied, Liars, Gossips

— Offender, Offended, Wounded, Healed

— Big nose, Small nose, Short, Tall, Wide, Thin

I think you get the picture! This book isn't about the things that we think define us, but they actually divide us if we let them define us. We talk about the importance of living in a diverse culture based on these things, and instead, they have become ugly divisions that bring bitterness, dissension, and hatred.

What this book is about are the things that are too priceless and too precious to be purchased, yet are so deeply desired and sought after by every human being under the sun, EVER.

Even in our differences, the common thing we share is that none of us are exempt from pain, grief, suffering, love, hope, gratitude, joy, happiness, and peace. It is not our circumstances that define us, but what we choose to do with them that will determine our course for this life, and how we will live it. Gratitude lightens our load because we allow others into our brokenness to help us with the burdens of this life, bringing joy, happiness, and peace. We must remember that bitterness divides, dissension and hatred destroy. Love wins ALWAYS and rebuilds hopes, dreams, and lives.

This true story will challenge and inspire you to let love and gratitude guide your heart, thoughts, and actions when it would be easier to bury your head in the sand. It is more than a feeling, it is a decision that needs to be made many times each day, namely, to choose to love in any and every situation.

In this collection of memories from so many family members and friends, you will see the scarlet thread of love in every chapter through Matt's blog that carefully stitched so many hearts together with a strength and beauty that brought shape and purpose to the fabric of Mary Kaye's healing and life.

It is our hope and prayer that as you read each word of every sentence written, that true love, pure love would enter your heart; that you would find hope, healing, refreshing, and a renewed purpose for your life. Let love win for you!

Love and blessings,

Mary Kaye (MK), Matt, and Brenda

Introduction

I coded (died) three times starting the evening of November 21 through early November 22, 2013. This is my story of coming back, of overcoming, of living, of love. Writing this book has been very emotional for me. I have asked my loved ones to relive the pain, fear, joy, hope, and darkness during a helpless time in our lives and our darkest hours. We have had conversations and shared memories from that time while I was hooked up on life support, not knowing what we would do from day to day. Even though we know the outcome of this traumatic experience, it is still very difficult for my family to live through again to be able to share it with you. I don't know how to adequately thank them for their time, then and now.

While in the process of trying to heal this anoxic brain injury—at least not give up trying—I would like to explain what it is like in hopes of helping you to understand what my "new normal" is. Perhaps, with this knowledge, you can overlook the typos, misspellings, and incomplete thoughts as I try to share our story.

One day, while Matt (my husband) and I were alone on the deck watching the clouds, I explained to him that I feel like my head is that way…it’s cloudy. Some days are rain clouds when I cry out of sadness. I experience feelings of being overwhelmed listening to a special song or a sad audiobook. But with the rain, there's always a rainbow! I am joyful for this opportunity to live yet another day for him, Aubrey, Emily, our family, and friends!

I do, however, look forward to days with no clouds, just sunshine and clear thoughts! That will be a special day when I can move freely and without hesitation or pain!

Matt reached for my hand and gently said, “I know your fear and hesitation. I understand looking back and trying to remember the freedom you once had, your old life. It won’t help. That part is gone and it’s up to you to find and embrace your new normal. Never stop. Never quit. Believe you are here for a reason. We are blessed with people who come our way with understanding, patience, and encouragement.”

He has taken on this journey with me, and he is my cheerleader, my confidant, and always my friend! I am so blessed! This is my story. I can’t force anyone to believe it, but it is my prayer that you will find hope.

CHAPTER 1

My Life in Pieces

"I spent last night" is the first line of what is still a very special song, but "I Spent Last Night In The Arms Of Jesus" should be my saving grace, is my saving grace!

I am Mary Kaye Decker Podschweit, and I was born on November 25, 1966, in Davenport, Iowa to Theodore and Karen Decker. I was the youngest of seven. I grew up in a tiny slab three-bedroom, one-bath home in Silvis, Illinois. I was the most loved of all the children...at least that's what I like to remind my siblings!

Life had its tragedies including the loss of two sisters, both in traumatic ways. One was lost to suicide and the other, well, she cut us out of her life. We learned about her passing by reading the obituaries.

Mom had her fair share of heartache. I have seen her at her lowest times in grief. Grief is an ugly mask. During this time, I witnessed God's love, grace, and joy as she struggled with her own pain. I think the thought of putting Mom through another death of one of her children, her last living daughter, was one of my motivating factors. I couldn't bear having her heart broken yet again.

Daddy's girl!

It's amazing what goes through your head and your heart when life is at its most fragile state. I miss my dad. He was a puzzle and I love puzzles.

One of my fondest memories of Dad was my sophomore year. The school office called me out of biology. I was scared, and wondering what I had done wrong. All the way to the office I was thinking, "Did I say something wrong, or cheat, or did the school decide to place me in a reading program because I stutter?" The stuttering got worse the more scared I became. I was preparing my rebuttal for the special class as I walked to the office. In grade school, when I worked with a speech therapist I was tormented by my classmates, which just made my speech that much worse. Even now, remembering those moments causes me great anxiety. As I approached the office, I was stunned to see my dad waiting for me. I thought that someone in our family may have gotten hurt and I began to cry.

Dad smiled and hugged me and whispered in my ear, "Let's go get some lunch." He signed me out and took me to Steak 'n Shake. We shared a strawberry shake with two straws and two spoons! He apologized for not being there for me and explained that he and Mom were in so much pain and that it had been difficult. The pain my dad shared with me was the loss of my sister, Barbara. After we had finished talking, we went to a sports store and he bought me new volleyball shoes.

My Sister Barbara

Barbara was beautiful in my eyes. She had light brown, naturally curly hair and bright blue eyes with very fair skin. She had a medium build and stood about 5'7." Her eyes seemed to express the sadness that she felt and the burdens that she carried unknown to everyone else. She lived in a silent heartache. She was the more caring of my sisters but was severely bullied at school. She was partially deaf from an accident when using a bobby-pin in her ear. It ruptured the eardrum which caused permanent hearing loss. This along with being poor made her an easy target. Barbara hated school but loved her teachers. The other girls in school were relentless about beating her up and making fun of her. They would take her lunch and throw it in the garbage...telling her that the garbage is where she needs to eat because she smells like a pig. One day the school had called (I was at home sick) and told my mom to come and pick up my sister. She was beaten pretty badly and the girls had given her a swirly by sticking her head in the toilet and flushing it. She didn't defend herself.

Not long after that, Barbara made the decision to drop out of school. I don't blame her. She met a young man named Bob, and they eloped when she was eighteen. Bob was a drug dealer and Barbara worked at Village Inn bussing tables.

My brother David and Dad tried very hard to get Barb to leave Bob. David even offered her all of his savings to help her leave but she was too afraid.

Early one Friday evening, I was at a friend's house. When Mom came to get me, I could tell that she had been crying. She told me that Barbara had called to see if she could have some money. Mom said that it sounded like Barbara had been crying, and Mom was feeling helpless. She told Barbara that she would help her if she would come home. Barbara explained that she thought she could leave Bob tomorrow. But tomorrow never came for her.

The story goes that, while at a bar in Bettendorf, Iowa, Bob demanded that Barbara give him all her money including her paycheck. She refused, so he beat her up in the bar, and then he forced pills down her throat. He finally got what he wanted—all of her cash and her paycheck. He then told her to go clean herself up. She went to the bathroom, locked the door, and crawled out of the window.

Naturally, being distraught, Barbara began walking *(I like to think she was walking home)*. She had to cross the I-74 bridge from Bettendorf, Iowa to Moline, Illinois, and then walk through East Moline to get to our home in Silvis. *(It truly seems like a stretch to believe that she was trying to get home but I take comfort in this.)* While walking on the bridge, against traffic, she stopped in the middle where there was a small landing, and there she stood. Traffic stopped. A police officer saw what was going on and made his way to her. They began talking. A crowd of people began to gather and then began chanting "JUMP- JUMP-JUMP!" The officer tried very hard to take her hand but she did what people were chanting...she jumped. The crowd cheered. They literally cheered her to her death. The officer was so shaken up he had to leave the force.

That night my brother Danny and I had fallen asleep in the living room when we heard a knock at the door. Danny opened it and there stood a pastor and two police officers. They asked for us to get our parents. I ran back and woke up Mom and Dad while Dan invited them in. It was that moment that changed our family dynamic forever. After that night, Dad became fiercely protective of us, and Mom just cried.

I believe it was a week later when they recovered her body from the Mississippi River, on a Saturday morning. Danny and I were watching "Hi Ho Silver" when a news story broke in and interrupted the program. It was a special report of the search and rescue team hauling my sister from the water. There were massive hooks in her body as they drug her to the shore. My oldest brother, Tommy was standing on the shoreline and the news broadcaster tried to ask him questions. He turned to look at the reporter, tears streaming down his face, and walked away. That picture still haunts me today. Barbara's death was deemed a suicide because her body was full of the drugs that Bob had shoved into her mouth, but no witnesses would come forward because he had threatened them. I only know this story because one of the men that was with my sister and Bob that night told me what had happened. I have no way of proving what was said, but I believe him because I want to.

I look for Barbara in strangers' faces, thinking about what she might look like today. I have found a few ladies that resemble what I picture her looking like, and have quickly shared my story with them and then ask them if I can take their pictures. I share them with my family. As difficult as her life was, she always had a smile for me! I have often asked God to punish everyone who was mean to my sister and the school who didn't do enough to protect her, and I have prayed that Bob would turn himself in.

I was eleven, and it was the summer before my seventh-grade year.

My Brother David

His first years he navigated living in a trailer with Mom, Dad, a brother, and two sisters. That's a lot of people to live in a trailer. When our parents purchased their first home and only home he was five years old. For his next birthday, he received the best present ever (at least I like to remind him of this), me! I was born on his birthday. He is six years older.

He is now 6'6" with an executive-style haircut! He is extremely handsome and we call him King Midas because everything he touches seems to turn to gold! David knows how to make people feel worthy and important—people always leave his presence feeling better about themselves. David was only seventeen years old when Barbara died and had the love to help take care of me. My parents were frozen—unsure of how to breathe some days. The "what-ifs" haunted my mother then, and I think even to this day. It was during this time in our family's life that my brother, David, whom I consider to be one of the greatest men in my life, began parenting me. He made sure I was enrolled in school, would talk to my teachers, and would always make sure that I had clean clothes to wear.

He is a great comforter and is always the first one to celebrate special moments!

My Brother Danny

Danny is 6'5—shorter than David, and it was always a point of teasing between them. He was a great athlete playing football and wrestling all through high school. Danny is very handsome; his eyes are shockingly baby blue. He was always very protective of me at school. He and David were the caretakers of our family after Barbara passed away. He is only seventeen months older than me but wise beyond his years or as Dad would tease, wise beyond his ears!

Dan is very, no scratch that, incredibly protective of all of us. Once he finds out that there is a need, he is always willing to help. He is always about finding a solution. He and his wife, Shelly, are two very generous people, kind-hearted and fun.

My Brothers Bill and Tom

Bill and Tom are very dear to me. We all handle grief in our own way. Losing Barbara the way we did has proven a very difficult path for all. I am thankful for the support and love they continue to provide.

I have decided to share my greatest struggles and victories. The good, bad, and the ugly which have given me the strength, the fight, the faith, and the belief that good comes from even the bad. After all, if our lives were always filled with sunny days we would live in a desert, so embrace the struggles and grow!

Me

As I entered seventh grade all my teachers were very empathetic and knew of my sister's death. I remember them all being so kind. Entering Junior High School was going to be hard, but then I made the volleyball team. I tried out for cheerleading but was the first cut. I tried out for cheerleading again in eighth grade. This time I was the second one cut, but then I made the volleyball team.

Some say cursed, others say blessed—nevertheless I was a busty 5'7" with blondish-brown hair and 130 pounds of awkwardness! When I went into high school, yup—you guessed it, I tried out for volleyball and was quickly moved up to JV. But this time I was an alternate cheerleader! I was your typical student just trying to navigate life and stay away from bullying. I had friends and we would buy cinnamon schnapps and go drinking before the football and basketball games. One game I got caught by one of the teachers that knew our family. He told me that my parents had gone through enough heartache so he wasn't going to call them. Instead, he called my brother David. David's disappointment in my decisions was both painful and hard-hitting.

Loss of Self

I graduated from high school in May of 1984 and began college that fall. I continued to play volleyball and made some spectacular friendships, some of which continue today! Zelda was one of them, and we became inseparable! She is a 6'1" blonde bombshell, funny, and sensitive! We began playing beach volleyball, grass and indoor volleyball leagues, and tournaments. Our friendship became a healing one for me. She would challenge me to always be better in the game, as a daughter, and a friend!

One weekend the AVP (American Volleyball Professionals) were playing in Chicago. We grabbed our girlfriends and drove the two hours to watch the tournament and got a nice hotel in walking distance to the beach! Off we went with our money, water, bagels, and apples!

We came across a group of young boys picking on a person who looked like he needed something to eat. He may have been a homeless man. He was dirty and lonely and was begging the boys to stop, but they just laughed. Zelda and I began talking to him, which was a great disappointment to the boys. They left to harass someone else, I am sure.

My heart was hurting, thinking of my sister Barbara. If someone would have seen her and helped her while she was being bullied, maybe just maybe she would have stayed in school, and if she would have stayed in school, maybe she would have never met Bob, the drug dealer. She could still be with us. My mind was a whirlwind of "what-ifs."

I gave the man my water, food, and money. I figured with Zelda's looks all of our needs would be taken care of! I wasn't trying to pimp out my friend but we were able to get an invitation to a private party where all the professional players would be! Come to find out, several teams were also staying in the same hotel that we were.

On our way back to the hotel after a successful day on the beach, we saw the same homeless guy. He was passed out leaning on the same tree where we first encountered him. In his hand was a brown paper bag with what appeared to be alcohol and next to him was my bag of bagels and apples. My heart hurt, not because he purchased alcohol with the money, but that he felt he had no other options than to drink. I have no explanation for how I felt; I knew I needed him to smile at me to let me know he was okay. But we walked away heavy hearted.

We showered and got dressed for the night out. Everything is always fun when we are together! We had developed quite the reputations amongst the volleyball community. We were referred to as the “NUNsters," simply because we had none, didn’t want none, and didn’t give none! Believe me, many guys tried but always came back rejected! I loved being a nunster. I thought I was safe.

While in the hotel lobby a cab was called to take us to the party. Several of the pros came down into the lobby as well. They took one look at my girlfriends and asked if they could join us. Zelda was not keen on this idea but our friend, Sexy Sylvia, insisted. So off we went six of us in one cab!

The party was great—free drinks and food! I became rather shy and wanted to leave. Sexy Sylvia was talking to one of the players and pointing at me. I began blushing, and I felt very uncomfortable. I told my friends I was going back to the room and I would see everyone when they got back. Zelda and Sexy Sylvia stayed after she convinced one of the players to go back and escort me to my room. This player was married and I knew him and his career—he was known on tour as “the good guy.” Feeling comfortable with this decision, we caught a cab and made our way back to the hotel. When I got back to our room, one of our friends was in the throes of entertaining and I couldn't go in. I said I would just wait in the lobby, and "the good guy" with me said he had a room all to himself; I could stay there until my room opened back up. That seemed like a better option than waiting in the lobby, so I agreed.

Innocence Lost

I remember his room being very clean and organized. His dirty clothes were in a separate suitcase, and his tournament clothes were laid out for the next day. I remember being impressed and sat down in a chair. I began feeling uncomfortable about being in his room and he sensed it. He asked me if I wanted something to drink. I said no and thanked him for his hospitality but said I would feel more comfortable waiting downstairs. He then motioned for me, wanting to show me something. I obliged. When I got up and started for him, he grabbed me and threw me up against the wall. His strength was difficult to handle, and I began to scream. He then flipped me around so my face was pressing against the wall, wrapped a towel around my mouth and tugged. He reached under my skirt and ripped my panties off. He told me not to scream, or he would hurt me. Then he entered me and pulled out to finish. He then demanded that I get undressed—I did. He turned on the shower and cleaned himself from between my legs. Any evidence of what had just happened was now down the drain.

All the while he was cleaning me he was reminding me how he is respected on the tour as "the good guy" and if I were to say anything no one would believe me. All of them would just hate me, after all, this is my fault. Said he wouldn't tell anyone in order to protect me. Once he dried me off, he told me to get dressed—I did. I don't know what happened to my underwear, but I put my bra, shirt, and skirt back on and slipped on my sandals. He did a quick inspection and then said, "It's our secret. I won't tell if you don't." I asked him if I could go, and all he said was "*Remember...*"

I ran back to our hotel room only to find our other roommate passed out with her friend, and both of them were naked. So, I grabbed my underwear and a jacket and left. I wandered the streets of Chicago in shock at what had just happened. I was too scared to say anything and doubtful that anyone would believe me. I went to where I last saw the homeless man and sat at his tree. The next thing I remember the sun was coming up, so I made my way back to the hotel. There I found Zelda and Sexy Sylvia, who had slept in the car because our room was occupied. I was able to wake my friends and we made our way to our empty room. I showered and scrubbed with hot water. My friends were ready to go back to the tournament, so I told them that I would meet them there.

When they left, I hopped back in the shower and scrubbed myself again until there was no more hot water. I could not get clean, and I cried like I had when I had lost my sister. I cried because my innocence was gone. I cried because I hated myself, and I cried because I blamed myself. I cried because I was alone.

Contemplating Living

Shortly after coming home from our Chicago trip, I went into a shell. My tears had dried, but my sense of self remained in tatters. I was numb. I didn't dwell in the past or look to the future. My family and friends, my loved ones, wanted me back, but no one knew what had happened. They couldn't. My light had been extinguished. I was in the dark alone, I had to be alone, barely there, finding it difficult to accept what had happened. I would be a different person from here on out. I didn't know how to breathe some days. I was unable to look at myself in the mirror, feeling alone with the words: "This is your fault. Everyone will hate you." The scary thing is, I believed him.

One day, feeling overwhelmed with those haunting words, I decided the pain was too much. The guilt was shameful. I couldn't see a light in this dark place. I was suffocating.

I felt at that time my only solution was to take my life, to take away the pain.

I composed a note to my family explaining this was not their fault and they would be okay without me. Never explaining why, too embarrassed even at death to tell them what had happened.

Willfully I made my way to the kitchen and grabbed an older knife from the drawer, purposely avoiding Mom's new kitchen knives. I then proceeded to numbly walk to the bathroom with the knife and my carefully, beautifully handcrafted note.

I grasped both a bath towel and a hand towel from the cabinet in our only bathroom. I took the time to attentively fold a hand towel and gingerly place it on a chair next to the tub. Gently kissing the note and carefully placing it on top of the towel. I then grabbed the bath towel to rest my slit wrist on. I wanted to make sure all this would be "easy." I would stay in the tub, avoiding a mess. I would try and keep everything neat and clean. Clambering into the bathtub fully dressed I lay down and cried. I cried like I had when I had lost my sister. I cried because my innocence was gone. I cried because I hated myself, and I cried because I blamed myself. I cried because I was alone.

I took the seasoned knife, a knife that had been used for celebrations, holidays, and making countless dinners, and deliberately began slitting my left wrist.

The blood was immediate. I lay there thinking, "Oh, God, what have I done!"

Images of my mom and dad came flooding through. The images of pain all these years after losing Barbara to suicide. Images of my brothers being mad at me, of Dan blaming himself for not being there, of David's disappointment. I didn't want to put those I loved through more anguish. What have I done?

"Oh God, please help me, please let me live!"

I grabbed the hand towel that I had placed near the tub and applied instant pressure. The knife was old and therefore not sharp enough to cut the vein but the cut was deep enough to leave a scar which I still have to this day. It's a reminder of a time in my life when God knew me, He pursued me, even when I didn't really know Him. He loved me even when I couldn't love myself.

A few months passed and Zelda and I were talking. She noticed my passion for playing volleyball and going out had diminished. I didn't want to play anymore, and I didn't want to go out. She thought she had done something, and with tears in her eyes, she said, "Please tell me what I have done so I can make up for it...apologize."

It was in that moment I gave in and spoke the words out loud. "I was raped," I told her everything. We both cried. At that time, I had decided I never wanted to be in a relationship or have children because the world is a cruel place. Over time Zelda got me back out on the volleyball court and around friends.

And This is Matt—My Friend, My Love!

You know when you first see someone and your soul begins to sing? That moment in time when your eyes meet and there's something so familiar and warm? That's the moment that I knew what I believed in would somehow change. I picked out everything wrong with him. I even made stuff up. I didn't want a relationship, and I certainly did not want to date a musician. Matt was a very accomplished piano player, and I swear there were always girls around him, although he will humbly say that they were there for another band member. As soon as he saw me no one else mattered. He knew he needed to meet me. No matter how hard I tried to stay clear of him, we always seemed drawn to each other like a magnet. He will freely admit that he never thought he would be with someone like me.

We began dating and he was a pure gentleman. He would often share with me that he was so afraid of scaring me off he would focus on things like opening all doors, holding my hand, and insisting on paying for everything (*the dirty rat)*! When we started to become intimate, I would pull away. The images of what happened in Chicago would surface because the man who raped me had been known as a gentleman. I didn't trust. I couldn't.

Matt had called me and asked me out for lunch. I was hesitant but he persisted. We then talked, my heart was heavy. I was in love with this beautiful and compassionate man who didn't deserve my harsh treatment. So I took a deep breath and told him what had happened. It's only the second time I had shared the words, "I was raped."

My head was down, and there were tears running down my face. When I finished telling him the story, I looked up to see this very talented, very beautiful man crying. He asked if he could hold my hand. I shook my head yes. He reached across the table and gently caressed my hand and said, "This was not your fault, this was not my fault. Don't hate US, because we are something special and I will never hurt you." I cried out, "But I am scared! I'm broken. I never wanted a relationship and I don't want a family. I don't want to bring anyone into this world. It's cruel!"

He stared at me with a puzzled look on his face and asked, "Am I cruel?" I cried, "No, not you, but people are and how can I bring anyone I love into my pain?" I said it. I said the word, "love." Matt was taken back by those words and his pain turned into joy! He said, "I love you and we will find a way!"

The Ted Talk: Matt's perspective

I knew from day one of meeting Mary that I wanted her to be mine forever. Something about her smile drew me in and like a moth to light, I couldn't get enough.

Meeting her parents, Karen and Ted, for the first time was odd, actually. Ted probably weighed one hundred pounds and was on oxygen. He was supposed to be on oxygen all of the time, but he wouldn't quit smoking. When he wasn't smoking, he was sleeping. He couldn't stop or wouldn't stop smoking the unfiltered Pall Malls. He was salty! I thought of him as frail until he went to shake my hand. Wow! His grip was so tight! For a man that looks so sick, MAAAN was he strong! His nicotine-stained fingers wrapped around my hand and he told a joke as he shook my hand rather aggressively.

Laughter! He loved to make people laugh. We quickly became friends. I would often go pick him up to go out for a hamburger but Ted was an avid golfer, a sport I never tried until I wanted to ask Mary to be my wife.

One day in early February, I asked if he wanted to go to the indoor driving range. He laughed so hard and said, "Yes, but don't tell Karen, she thinks we always go to the strip club!" We got to the driving range and everyone knew him. It was like walking into the TV show *Cheers* when everyone says, "Hey Norm!" He never knew a stranger. Since I was a novice golfer at best, Ted offered to show me a few things. He was trying to help me with my swing. His instructions were, "'Matt, point your left foot toward the hole and take your right foot and point it towards the clubhouse. Keep your head down and swing that club!"

I did what he said, and when I swung I did hit the ball, about three feet, and my legs buckled and I fell on the green! Embarrassed I look up to see Ted laughing so hard he was crying!

We had a beer. Well, I had a beer. Ted had a container of salt with some beer. I then asked him if I could marry his daughter. He said, "I couldn't imagine a better son-in-law."

CHAPTER 2

This Is Us

Matt is the most caring man I have ever met. He proposed on February 25, 1992, and we began planning our wedding for Labor Day weekend that same year! Then I became pregnant. Remember, I didn't want children. We did a good job of ensuring that would never happen. But the best-laid-out plan always has a ripple, so we decided to move the wedding to June 27, 1992.

My lack of happiness did not suppress Matt's overwhelming joy of becoming a father! Every day he would lay his head on my lap and sing to my growing tummy the same song over and over by one of his favorite musicians, Harry Connick Jr. As the baby grew, she would move when she heard Matt begin to sing "I'll Dream of You Again." As he began singing the beginning of this beautiful song "I spent last night dreaming of your eyes," she would press against my ever-growing tummy. It was extraordinary!

Aubrey Kathryn

On October 23, 1992, we became parents to a beautiful daughter, Aubrey! I thought I knew love by being with Matt but once the doctor placed our girl in my arms and we caught eyes, I knew a different kind of love! She began to fuss and then Matt began singing our song and she cooed! The song brought great comfort then, and it still does!

On December 17, 1992, my dad passed away. But before he did, Matt and I made our way to the hospital to see him. We walked into his room and Dad said, "You're having another baby?" I replied, "No, Dad, we just had Aubrey a few months ago." He smiled and said, "I know, but you are going to have another child." Those were his last words to us.

Emily Grace

As we were figuring life out I became pregnant again. And once again Matt would sing to my growing belly "I spent last night dreaming of your eyes, but your hair kept getting in the way, your lips dropped in...," and again our second child, Emily, would respond in the same way as Aubrey did! The girls are only sixteen months apart and I jokingly told Matt he couldn't look at me without us getting pregnant so he had a vasectomy.

Our sweet Emily was very sick with kidney disease for the first seven years of her life and endured thirteen surgeries. It seemed that we were always at the hospital in Pediatric ICU. Aubrey would always be whisked away by family because the hospital would never allow her to be near Emily. We took turns at the hospital so that she would never be alone. We never knew the impact that had on Aubrey until she was asked to speak at a hospital fundraiser. She shared how difficult it is to love someone, a sister, that you may not have with you tomorrow. During that time, Aubrey learned how to be empathetic, and Emily learned to be competitive. It's Emily's competitive spirit that got her to where she is today and the fight she has for those she loves. Aubrey's empathetic spirit helps her navigate hard times.

New Faith

Our lives together brought many highs and lows. We moved my mom with us from Silvis, Illinois to Eureka, Illinois for a new job. Matt had been raised Lutheran and I was a "Chreaster" (Christmas and Easter believer). We were invited to attend a church service by Matt's boss, Dave; our insurance agent, John; and a speaker named Larry. Mom was also invited to church by her new co-worker, Sharon. We joked about attending all these churches and decided to go to Dave's church first.

When we walked in the doors of that small country church, Congerville Mennonite, we were greeted by Dave, John, Larry, and Sharon! Everyone was so happy to see us and they all thought we were there from their invite! There was no way we would ever say we were only there because Matt's new boss invited us! There was something familiar and so genuine about walking through those doors that morning. Matt shared after our visit to the Mennonite Church that he would like the girls to have a Christian upbringing and I agreed. So Sundays became a family day! Mom has always been a strong believer and made great friends through the church, and now Matt and I were finding our way.

On Easter 1996, Matt came home from a men's breakfast and shared with us that he had had an epiphany and that Jesus must be real because at that moment Matt made a conscious effort to ask "Why?" instead of "Why not?" A week later I understood, and we were baptized together in a special service! Zelda drove down to celebrate this special time with us!

Whenever there was a stressful time, Matt would sing our song to me! "I spent last night dreaming of your eyes but your hair kept getting in the way. Your lips dropped in to tell me how you'd been but when I tried to kiss them..." He would hold my hand and kiss me gently on my head until I was able to sleep. When the girls were sick he would always hold them and they would ask him to sing. No matter how he tried to sneak in a funny VeggieTales song they would end up with "I spent last night..."

Coaching

I had decided to sneak into Eureka High School to watch the girls' volleyball practice. I was standing in the doorway appreciating the beauty of the gym. The team strategically moves in unison with the ball. That's one thing I love about the game…it's the dance! It's like a beautiful choreography of six people and an animated coach. The head coach saw me, waved and proceeded to come over. Coach Kary Cram is a young, kind, vibrant, math teacher who loves volleyball like I do! She asked if I knew anyone there. I said, "No, I am just watching." Coach Cram then invited me into the gym and asked me to scrimmage with the girls and coaches. I must have been beaming! I was doing something I loved and finding the fire that was lit back in seventh grade! It was so fun and everyone was so nice! Coach asked if I could give her setters a few tips, so I did, and the girls responded and adjusted quickly. Coach asked if I could come to practices to help out. I explained I had two young girls at home, and she said, "Would they help shag balls?" I smiled and said that they would love that! The team adopted Aubrey, Emily and me! I coached at Eureka High School and Middle School until 2003.

Call of Ministry

One time, when visiting the Quad Cities, our good friend, Scott Schaefer, told Matt he would serve the church someday. In 2003, Matt accepted a position with Heritage Wesleyan Church in Rock Island, Illinois (the church where Scott served on staff). So, we all moved back to the Quad Cities, and we were there for six years! Six amazing years of being wrapped in the arms of wonderful, loving people who became friends! Matt had a whirlwind European trip with our missions pastor Rich Lively where he made more friends from the Czech Republic, Croatia, Poland, and Germany. Our life was good!

During our time in Rock Island, Matt didn't have a reason to sing our song to me. We adopted other family things. Our favorite was every VeggieTales song, game night, and entertaining.

In July of 2010, we moved to Colorado to be closer to Matt's mom Judy and his sister Rhoni, her husband Dave, and our two nieces Alex and Kennedy. We have always lived close to my family; there was no way I would ever deny Matt his wish!

Matt began working for USA Volleyball in 2011. The girls were state champs with their high school volleyball teams. The transition was smooth. Aubrey had a few Division II schools recruiting her and Emily had a few Division I schools pursuing her. Emily's heart was beach volleyball, which helped her indoor game greatly! Aubrey began her college career at Regis University in Denver and Emily received a generous beach volleyball scholarship in Florida. I was so happy—we were a volleyball family!

CHAPTER 3

Where There are Geese...There is Poop!

November 20, 2013

Matt and I were excited about coaching a twelve and under girls' volleyball team together, and our daughter Aubrey was going to be the club's setting coach! The girls and their parents were both excited and scared about the season. The talk with the parents is always difficult because everyone wants their child to be a star...and guess what? I am quite good at making everyone feel special! My job was to allow these girls to fall in love with the game!

The first day of practice is my favorite day of the season, and the first practice sets the tone for the season! On this morning, I was thinking about volleyball practice and developing a practice plan in my head. I was already setting into motion a game plan.

We love to start with get-to-know-you games by playing "Red Rover, Red Rover, send those whose favorite color is red over!" We make games out of things from pet hamsters to how many siblings you have. My absolute favorite game is "Hot Potato" to work on reactionary skills! Laughter always ensued. If you need to know one thing about me, it is that I love to laugh!

I was out walking early that morning and the air had a crisp November chill. About 200 yards away was a water feature. The fountain in the middle of the man-built pond was very serene. The mountains had a beautiful snow-cap and the sun was gleaming in the blue sky. The moment was very surreal, so instantly charming. My mind began to wonder, how the pioneers must have felt seeing America's mountain which we call Pikes Peak. Sheer curiosity!

That time of year Canadian Geese were still migrating. The water feature, I can only imagine, was a great spot for a break for the geese. They can be loud and aggressive if you are not careful. This is why I was carefully navigating my walk, staying as far away from them as possible while still admiring the beauty of the birds and the snow-capped mountains in the crispness of the morning.

Naturally, along with so many geese, as you can imagine, is an amazing amount of goose poop. I stepped on a fresh pile of this disgusting source of natural excrement and slipped! I didn't fall but caught myself.

The embarrassment of slipping was laughable. Red in the face, I balanced myself and gingerly began to walk to my destination. The pain was immediate and intense. “Great!” I thought, “I just broke my left ankle.”

I am certain that while you are reading this you are thinking, “How did she not see the poop?” That seems to be everyone’s unyielding question when I tell this story.

In all fairness, I was distracted that morning. You see, I had just been in a fender bender. I happened to be making a left turn and began pulling out into the intersection and the car behind me decided to go and ram the back end of my car. Okay, it was more of a tap than a hit...but still, it was very alarming!

We both pulled over. The man got out of his car and he looked pissed, red in the face—mad! It scared me. He came up to the driver’s side and knocked on the window, motioning me to roll down my window. I hesitantly did what he requested. When he stared at me I realize he was a dwarf. Standing on his tiptoes he barely reached the bottom of my window. His glare was intense. He puts his hands on his hips and said in a deep voice like a character from Snow White, “I’m not Happy!” It sent a shiver up my spine. All I could do was look at him and respond in my most sarcastic tone, “Well, which one are you?”

Of course, that never happened! I was never in a fender bender anyway—I did, however, slip on goose poop!

I called my daughter Aubrey, and she came and got me in her old, broken-down van that we affectionately called Goldie. We made our way to the emergency room. I was feeling rather stupid and quite embarrassed as I was wheeled back to x-ray. I could hear the beeping from the other patient's rooms, and it made me sad. I wondered:

What are their stories?

Do they have family with them?

Are they going to be okay?

And the babies who were crying...I was flooded with emotions thinking of the countless times we were in the emergency room with Emily. Panic was rearing its ugly head, and I wanted to go so badly so that I didn't take time away from those who really needed care. I wanted to be okay, to get up and walk and leave. Not that I felt I didn't deserve the care but so many people were there asking for help.

Aubrey was a wonderful counselor to me at that moment. She explained that if it was a break or a sprain, it was still good that I was there. The doctor would come with a game plan and once he did, then we could go. She then assured me that if someone came in with an urgent need they would care for them before finishing up with me, "because an urgent medical crisis is real and if we were in urgent need, they would make us a priority." Such wise words that would be truer in twenty-four hours. I would be that patient who needed immediate medical assistance!

The diagnosis was a high sprain. The doctor's orders were to keep weight off the foot with the use of crutches, to take pain meds, and to see an orthopedic doctor on November 22.

Aubrey

Mom called me and asked if I could take her to the emergency room because she thought she broke her ankle. It's not like I don't have a life to figure out, so with a desperate sigh, I said I would be right over.

She was so cheerful, always so cheerful. She could tell by my lack of enthusiasm I was not pleased in having to take her. She tried desperately to make up for it by telling me one of her quirky jokes and funny stories. I knew if I would only laugh she would just be silent. But I couldn't. I didn't want to give her the satisfaction of knowing it was okay.

We got to the emergency room and they put her immediately in a private room. Mom now second-guessed the importance of being here. I literally rolled my eyes, and thought to myself, *"Why does she have to be like this? Always putting others first when it's rather obvious from the swelling and her degree of pain that she needs to have it looked at."*

Mom started compiling reasons to leave: others are in need, she doesn't want to distract from people who really need attending to, and so on and so on. I couldn't take it anymore and reached for her hand. "Mom," I said, "this is an emergency room; if someone needs to be seen before you they will. Relax." Now that I think about that day I feel rather ashamed. My empathy went right out the window along with my patience.

I then asked her about the game plan for her volleyball team. (I am reminded that is ANOTHER thing I really don't care to do but I do it because I know it makes her happy. Lord God give me the strength and grace that I need to love her.)

I tried to control my disappointment not only with her clumsiness but also with my lack of ability to tell her no. I could not wait to get her home so I could let off some steam and go have a drink with friends. There was no way I was going to babysit Mom until Dad got home. He could take care of her and her demands.

Finally, they came in to take her back for an x-ray. I had a chance to step outside and fill Dad in. The doctor came back rather quickly and said "I have good news. It's not broken but a rather high sprain. She will need to stay off of it and see an orthopedic doctor in the next few days." He prescribed pain meds and we were off. Next stop was to fill her prescription and then home. Finally.

Thank goodness Dad came home early and he helped me with her from the van to bed. And then I left. Just left. Never said goodbye or I love you. I left. I stayed over at a friend's house because I didn't want to help with Mom. Dad said she would be going back to work and asked if I could simply give her a call during the day to check on her.

I said, "Of course, Dad,"...but never did. I never called.

Emily

I called Mom every day walking from beach volleyball practice to the athletes' study hall at Florida International University in Miami, Florida. Sometimes I needed her to listen and other times I needed her to laugh. Pretty much I needed her. I had learned early on that the way to love my mom is at a distance. I am certain that every mother and daughter go through some kind of love-hate relationship. For me, I was fortunate enough to live in California for the summers since I was sixteen, and it was there that I began focusing on this very moment of my life, being a collegiate athlete and playing beach volleyball.

But with the struggles of independence at sixteen, I needed something to ground me and that was Mom's smile. I missed her smiling at me. It was always the first thing that came to mind when I thought of her on a daily basis, her smile. Not only her grin but her eyes! Yes, somehow they twinkled; I don't know if it was a mischievous look or a kind, loving look, or a combination of both, but she always managed a smile!

On November 20 Mom shared her story of slipping on goose poop and then followed with her seven dwarves joke. She was always trying to bring humor and provoke a laugh. Actually, I laughed so hard, I had to share that with my team! She was awesome at finding humor in the little things.

CHAPTER 4

Brokenness Begins

November 21, 2013

Matt arranged his schedule to take me to work and I certainly didn't mind the extra help especially from my very handsome chauffeur! I was feeling discouraged and still trying to find a rhythm with the use of the crutches; certainly not very graceful, rather dangerous actually. I am not the most graceful person on the planet, so to put me on a pair of crutches seemed rather ridiculous. The movement was not a flow of one sound with the crutches striking the ground at the same time, it was more like I was hobbling awkwardly! *Clip, shuffle, swing, clip, shuffle, stop, rearrange the crutches to be more comfortable. Clip, shuffle, swing, clip.*

Matt got me settled in my cubicle and as comfortable as he could make me. He looked around as to how to keep my foot elevated as best as possible. Being clever, he turned my recycle bin upside down and placed my back pillow over it. It was the best we could do with what we had.

The pain was becoming very intense. I didn't bring any pain pills with me and Tylenol and Advil were not doing much.

Working on balancing my accounts, trying diligently to ease my mind from the throbbing pain I did not get up from my desk all day, not even to use the bathroom. I sat there for nine hours. My coworkers often checked on me and did all they could to help me navigate my work. I could feel my leg beginning to swell and my pants became very tight around the leg. The pain was increasing. Alarmed but not panicked, I buried my head into balancing accounts, my work.

When Matt came to get me, he was concerned with how much pain I was in. Rather gingerly, he helped me to my feet and assisted with the agonizing, painfully slow progress to the car.

Clip, shuffle, swing, clip, shuffle, stop, rearrange the crutches to be more comfortable. Clip, shuffle, swing, clip.

That evening we were having our very first club volleyball team practice. The girls were age twelve and under and all so excited! Our first parent/player meeting had been held two weeks earlier at the Olympic Training Center in Colorado Springs. This would have been Matt's first year coaching. He's been to so many tournaments and games and has been with the top coaches in the country (a benefit of working for USA Volleyball). Matt has traveled the country going to both indoor and beach volleyball events. He was looking forward to the coaching aspect of his job! I have had the pleasure of yelling at kids for many years! Okay, you say coaching...yelling...same thing!

Once home, Matt helped me to the bathroom where I was able to relieve myself and change into comfortable clothing. The swelling was up my leg like I had suspected. We decided that our daughter Aubrey would help coach that night and give me some much-needed rest. It was painful, but he propped me up in a recliner and made me as comfortable as possible. Then he and Aubrey proceeded to leave once he felt like I had everything I needed. He made sure my phone was charged in case I needed anything and he promised that he would keep his on.

Aubrey

I came home around 5:15 p.m. on November 21 only to get my stuff ready for coaching volleyball. Mom was not going to make it and wanted to share with me the practice plan since it was Dad's first year. I didn't even take the time to listen.

Dad had her propped up in the recliner. She was in obvious pain, but dammit, how in the hell did she not see the goose poop? I got into the car and waited for Dad. Although I was extremely disappointed in my own reactions, I was not ready to reach out to offer any more help than what was required.

Emily

I stepped outside of my tutoring session on the night of November 21. I had tried calling Mom earlier after practice, but she did not answer the phone. The sky was so incredible with hues of blue, peach, pink, and orange. So peaceful. The palm trees on campus had a slight sway. The tall ornate grasses were dancing rhythmically as the sun was getting tucked away. Paradise! Mom would love being here.

Aubrey

When we got to practice, of course, Dad had a question that I could not answer. If only I had taken the time to listen. Sigh. Dad had to call home to ask Mom a question that I should have been able to answer. We were only at practice for five minutes and we couldn't handle it without her. She was always great at reassuring people. Yet, she didn't answer. He called again right away. By this time, he looked rather alarmed, and after a brief conversation he told me, "Something is wrong with your Mom; we have to get home."

Dad talked to the lead coach and explained that something didn't seem right and he and I would need to leave right away. No questions asked.

Me

While sitting in the recliner, legs outstretched and feet up, I had my phone charged and on—Matt had made sure of it. Our youngest daughter Emily called me. She was a sophomore on a beach volleyball scholarship at Florida International University. She was checking on me and how I was faring with the sprain. I told her I wasn't feeling well and the swelling had gone up my leg and it felt warm. Emily sounded concerned and said, "Mom, if it is the same leg as the ankle sprain, that sounds like a blood clot. You better get to the hospital." I assured her I was seeing the doctor in the morning and would be sure to mention it then. I have no other memory of our conversation.

Emily

Mom finally answered after a couple of attempts of trying to reach her. When I called Mom the night of November 21 she sounded like she was in pain. Not really focusing on her issues, I just wanted to check in. I had to study for exams. Yet, something in her voice alarmed me.

She explained that the pain was intense from her ankle sprain and the swelling had gone up her leg and felt hot. Concerned, I asked, "Mom, this is the same leg as the ankle sprain?" I already knew the answer but was looking for confirmation. "Yes," she said in a soft whisper. "That sounds like a blood clot, you better get to the hospital," I said with some urgency but not demanding.

Mom assured me she was seeing the doctor in the morning and would be sure to mention it then. Fair enough, I thought to myself. Although I was concerned, I finished studying, packed up my books, and went to a friend's house who lived close to the sand courts on campus. My phone was off and I went to bed.

Matt

I had several questions about the team meeting and Aubrey was not able to answer but I knew Mary would be able to satisfy the curiosity of the parents. I am sure another coach would have been able to answer but I felt an urgency to call her. Something in my heart was unsettled. I hated leaving her at home alone and in obvious pain, although she shushed us and promised she was okay. When I called the first time she didn't pick up, so I persisted and called again. When she answered she sounded distressed. I immediately told another coach we had to leave. I grabbed Aubrey and rushed home, not understanding the urgency but knowing and following my heart. The neurologist explained that it was that decision that snowballed into many quick decisions that saved her life.

I cannot tell you, I have no explanation for this immediate decision or this feeling of urgency other than God whispering to go and that is what we did.

When we bolted through the door, maybe ten minutes from the initial phone call, Mary was grabbing her chest and in a lot of pain. Her phone had fallen. I think she was trying to call for help but couldn't manage to complete the call.

Aubrey rushed to her side and I called 911. When the paramedics arrived I was in the process of moving the furniture out of the way. Mary was still in the recliner, half curled in the fetal position in obvious pain. She began losing consciousness and became dead weight. It took all the strength they had to lift her—three strong, young men, and they were working fast. They were able to do a quick evaluation and rushed her to the ER. Aubrey and I initially thought it was a heart attack. Scared, we hopped in the car ready to follow the ambulance but we were blocked in by the emergency vehicle in the driveway and had to wait. During our wait, I began praying and counseling Aubrey. The fireman who was at the house to assist didn't give us any encouragement or insight into what was happening. He only told us which hospital.

We arrived at St. Francis Hospital Emergency Department where they escorted us to a private waiting room. They shared at that time we would have to wait while they were evaluating Mary. I insisted on being with her, not wanting her to be alone, but the nurse was firm. "We will come and get you as soon as we can, but until that time you must stay here." We had no idea my loving wife was fighting for her life. Fighting to live.

Aubrey

I wasn't ready to see Mom in so much pain. She was in the same recliner that we had left her in grabbing her chest, crying, gasping for air, and trying to tell us she couldn't breathe. Her phone had dropped on the floor and she couldn't manage to pick it up. I reached for her, and said over and over again, "Mom, I am so sorry, I am so very sorry." Then, I heard Dad on the phone with 911. It seemed like they were there in an instant.

Dad began moving furniture aside so the paramedics had better access to reach Mom. Her breathing became labored and shallow. I was watching her die and all I could say was "I'm sorry."

It took three grown men to pick her up and place her on the gurney. She was not responding but they found a weak pulse. We received no assurances from any of the first responders or the fire department. One of the firemen told Dad they were taking Mom to St. Francis Hospital. That was all that was said, no comforting words or affirmation that it would be okay.

I have never felt so bad, so undeserving of love or forgiveness. When we arrived at the hospital, Dad and I were sent to a private waiting room. A part of me just wanted to believe that Mom was being dramatic and she would come in to greet us and say "Are you ready to leave because I want to go home."

Dad had tried calling Emily a few times by now and it kept going to voicemail. He asked me to track her down.

Suddenly, a **CODE BLUE** was announced over the speakers, and a nurse shouts through the door of the private waiting room where we were, "Is it okay to do chest compressions?" We were stunned into silence, and the nurse asked the same question more frantically! Then Dad immediately understood what was happening. "*YES!*" he cried out.

A few minutes later a doctor came out and explained that we should go talk to Mom. Although she was unconscious, he thought it would be best for her to hear our voices.

It was Dad's turn first. I don't remember what he said or if Mom could even understand him through the sobs. I didn't know what to say and all I could do was whisper in Mom's ear, "I'm sorry, so sorry, please don't leave me."

The doctor explained Mom needed an x-ray of her chest. They were ruling out a heart attack and were thinking it might be blood clots in her lungs but needed some more testing to confirm. They asked us to go back to the waiting area and would come and get us when we could see her again. As Dad and I stepped aside, they had begun rolling Mom down the hallway. She started coding again! A doctor jumped up on the cart and yelled if it was okay to begin chest compressions. Dad was in shock and was only able to nod and whisper, "Yes." **CODE BLUE** was again out on the speaker system!

Seven minutes of fear and believing Mom was dead! Dad and I collapsed into each other's arms! The emergency room doctor came in and explained they were able to get a weak pulse and were doing everything they could to stabilize her enough to get to ICU. He then asked us to reach out to family.

Matt

The first time she coded an ER nurse came flying into the room to get permission to do chest compressions. I was taken back by this request and yelled "YES," as **CODE BLUE** was announced over the intercom.

We began making calls, first to my mom and sister. They lived within a few hours and I know Mary would want them to be with us. When trying to call Emily, it went directly to voicemail. I hung up. What was I supposed to say?

Once they were able to get her heart beating again they sent for both of us. Mary had been coughing up blood. They didn't know if this was from her stomach or lungs but they ruled out a heart attack.

In disbelief of what had just happened Aubrey and I whispered love and encouragement as she lay there unable to respond. The doctors explained they needed a chest x-ray and would come and get us once the procedure was over.

While they began wheeling her out of the room and we were being escorted to the waiting room, my wife, my friend, my love went into cardiac arrest for the second time in front of Aubrey and me.

They pulled us to the side and brought her back into the room. The doctor straddled her and began chest compressions for the second time. The outlook was not good. We stood outside her room watching the emergency room staff work frantically yet calmly to get a pulse. We were escorted back to the waiting room. I did not want to leave her side but had no choice. **CODE BLUE** was again announced over the intercom.

Seven agonizing, tormenting minutes went by and the doctor came in to talk to us. He explained that they were able to get a pulse but it was weak. He then encouraged us to call family. He explained they were working on her for preparation to ICU.

He asked us again to talk to her. We whispered encouraging words through distraught tears of panic and were once again escorted out.

I had tried to call Emily again, but it went directly to voicemail. I knew I needed Aubrey to think of something other than my mom and what she just witnessed. I put her in charge of finding Emily and getting a flight to bring her home. I called David, Mary's brother. I tried to tell him what was going on but couldn't stop crying. He said they would be on the next flight out.

Judy (Matt's mother)

Matt called that night. In a hoarse voice, he was able to share that Mary was in ICU and it didn't look good. I asked if he wanted me to come down and there was silence. I simply said "Honey, I am on my way. Which hospital again?" Matt whispered, "St. Francis."

Rhoni (Matt's sister)

Mary and I were not close but had love and respect for each other. I think this is important to share because during everything that transpired over the next few months I saw a side of her that was remarkable.

Matt called me the evening of November 21. When I answered, it was difficult to understand, to listen between the tears of anguish. When I got out of him that Mary was at St. Francis Hospital and it was not good, I simply asked, "Do you want me to come over?" Tears flowing, my older brother was reaching out to me, asking me to be with him, not knowing or understanding how difficult the next twenty-four hours would be. He was finally able to say, "Yes." I told him I was on my way.

I called our Dad who lives in Batavia, Illinois, and shared with him the little I knew. I wasn't expecting his response. He said he and June would leave immediately. Dad, our very conservative father, was going to be here to do all he could to help. This was very reassuring.

Matt had already called Mom and she was in her car driving down to Colorado Springs. We arrived at the hospital at the same time. Mary was being checked into ICU.

Ron and June (Matt's dad and stepmom)

Rhoni called the evening of November 21. She was upset and explained that Mary was in the hospital and had already coded once. She and Judy were on their way to Colorado Springs. I asked if she thought it would be best for us to fly out. Immediately she said, "Yes, Matt and Aubrey need all of us."

We made our way to Midway Airport. June was calling flights. It didn't look like we were going to be able to fly out with the ice storm. Fortunately, there was a small window of opportunity and we were able to catch the next flight out.

David and Carla (Mary Kaye's brother and sister-in-law)

Matt called on the night of November 21, 2013. It was out of the ordinary for him to call. I initially thought he was in town for work. When I answered, Carla and I were winding down from our day. I never expected to hear the news that Mary was in the emergency room with a possible heart attack. It doesn't run in our family. Nothing was making sense, and it was difficult to determine what was being said, but I knew Matt was in distress.

I asked if Mom knew yet. He shared that he was trying to contact all immediate family and the next call was to Dan, then Mom. He did not want Mom to be alone when he called. I told him I thought that was a good plan. I offered to call but Matt insisted that he should call.

I asked him if we should fly out and without hesitation, he said, "Yes, I need you here, Mary needs you." He shared she was in St. Francis Emergency Room. No news if they would move her or if she would survive.

Carla and I booked an emergency flight out to Colorado Springs.

Emily

A few hours later a friend came to find me. He looked panicked. He told me my sister, Aubrey, was trying to get ahold of me. Just the sound of "my sister is trying to get ahold of me" set me in an awful panic. Selfishly, I was scared to return her call. I looked at my phone and saw several missed calls from Dad and Aubrey. It was that moment, that very moment, that everything changed.

I took a deep breath and called Aubrey back. I fell on my knees crying as she shared Mom was in the hospital and things were not looking good. "Mom, not Mom!" Dad was on the phone talking to Uncle David and Aunt Carla, and I could hear him crying. I wanted to be home. Aubrey had room on her credit card and booked me the first flight out.

I called my coach and let her know what was happening. She wanted to make sure I had everything I needed to get to the airport and assured me she would inform the team and my professors. I don't remember packing a bag or how I got to the airport.

My flight from Miami to Denver, Colorado had a layover in Chicago, Illinois. I was caught in an ice storm. It was two in the morning, and I was all alone and scared. I tried calling Dad but it went directly to voicemail. I just needed to hear it was okay, that it was a false alarm. Dad had tried calling when I was on the flight and his voicemail was just of him sobbing. I don't believe he intended to leave me that message. I was hoping it was tears of joy.

When I finally got ahold of Aubrey, she didn't say much, just, "Please be safe and Aunt Rhoni will be picking you up." Then she hung up. All alone with my thoughts, I went to Facebook to see if anything was being posted. Aubrey's status came up first. It simply said, "Please pray for my mom, we are in the emergency room and it's not good." That was the last post at 6:30 p.m. No updates. No answers.

Matt

Aubrey was now on the phone with Emily, so I made my next call to Dan and Mary's mother, Karen. Mary's Dad,

Ted, passed away many years ago and I didn't want Karen to be alone when I called her. Dan listened as the panic in my voice was uncontrollable. He left right away to go to Karen's. He wanted to be there when I called her. He assured me that he and Karen would fly out right away. When I called Karen, Dan had just walked through the door. All I remember is Karen saying, "Not Mary, not my little girl!"

Dan (Mary Kaye's brother)

I received an unexpected phone call from Matt and was alarmed by the panic in his voice. The dreadful news about Mary was gut-wrenching. I would do anything to take back his words of despair, of pain, of fear which engulfed me. What about Mom?, I thought. When he shared what was going on with Mary, and asked if Mom and I could come out right away, I knew it was serious. I asked him if Mom knew already. He told me that he wanted me to be there with Mom when he called, knowing that it would be very hard on her.

It's no secret that I hate to fly. Matt asked me to fly out with Mom, who is wheelchair-bound. I knew I would need help. I called my wife Shelly. She's always a quick thinker; she managed the itinerary and helped navigate the emergency flight, car rental, and hotel stay all while out of town for work. While Shelly was working on her end, I helped Mom pack a bag and enough medicine for a short stay. Mom was going to need extra care both physically and emotionally. Shelly sent out an immediate prayer request and I loaded Mom up in the car and we drove gingerly to the airport.

I kept reassuring Mom that Mary was a fighter. She would pull through. She would find a way.

Karen (Mary Kaye's Mom)

I wasn't expecting Dan at my door. When he came over I knew something was wrong. Then the phone rang. Dan said, "Mom, you need to answer that." It was Matt on the other end of the phone. He asked if Dan was with me. I calmly said he was. Then he told me what had happened. At this time Mary was still in the emergency room. My heart felt all alone. I wanted to be with her.

Dan and Shelly, Dan's amazing wife, had made arrangements for Dan and me to fly to Colorado. We were in the middle of an ice storm. I certainly wasn't thinking about safety or how my wheelchair would be an obstacle in traveling, I just needed to be with my precious girl. When we arrived at the airport they were canceling flights. Dan said we had better just stay here. I began to cry.

Dan talked to the airlines and explained our situation, but all flights were canceled from Moline due to the ice storm. I sat in the airport in deep grief. All I could do was to pray that God would spare my only living daughter. I asked if he could comfort her and give her the fight she would need to hang on.

Matt

Rhoni called our Dad and he and June made arrangements to come out immediately.

I sent out an immediate prayer request to everyone in my contact list, not anticipating how dark and frightening life was going to get, but knowing we needed friends to intervene for us at that moment. We were broken and scared. I contacted all the people I had met on my trip to Europe with Pastor Rich Lively, the volleyball community, people I had met on a plane, close friends, everyone and anyone who could lift us up in prayer.

Matt's Blog: Mary Kaye's Odyssey

Thursday, November 21, 2013

Posted November 22, 2013, 8:56 p.m. by Matthew Podschweit. [Updated December 1, 2013, 12:11 p.m.]

Mary Kaye began feeling light-headed and clammy at about 6:15 p.m. while she sat in the living room resting her sprained left ankle. Her symptoms intensified until sharp chest pains began—then I called 911 for an ambulance. Upon arrival at the emergency room, she began vomiting and blood was present, but not knowing whether it came from her lungs or her stomach, they sedated her and rushed to a CT scan. They found multiple tiny blood clots in both lungs. Then she crashed. The ER staff started CPR and sent for me and Aubrey. We stood outside her treatment room holding each other, bracing for the worst. They were able to get back a weak pulse, and told us we could see her. We whispered encouragement in her ear and each gave her a kiss, and then returned to the waiting room. A little while later, we were urgently summoned back to her treatment room as they were resuscitating her for the second time, with the suggestion that preparing goodbyes might be in order. They were able to bring her back again, and shortly thereafter, they were able to stabilize her enough to move her to a room in the ICU.

CHAPTER 5

Storms

November 22, 2013

Matt

They were able to stabilize Mary in order to go to ICU. Emily was en route. Everything that needed to be done was being done. All family that I was able to touch base with were on their way.

I was broken. Aubrey was broken. Judy Murphy, my mother, and Rhoni Hirst, my sister, drove from up north in Colorado. They met Aubrey and me in ICU. The four of us were in Mary's ICU room; she was on life support. The doctor was explaining that Mary had a pulmonary embolism, blood clots to the lungs. They had given her a drug that is only used in emergencies because of its toxicity, TPA. At this moment she was stable but no guarantees. Then alarms started sounding and the doctor jumped on her bed, straddling her as he is asking for permission to resuscitate.

That was the third time of coding. How much more could her body withstand of this violent but life-saving procedure? I wasn't sure how our lives would change from my decision to continue trying but I believed it was the right thing to do. I never second-guessed. I had to find faith and trust that somehow everything would be okay.

The four of us were rushed out of the room, out of the way. We all collapsed on the floor just outside her room, distraught, in tears, in grief. The intercom once again repeated, **CODE BLUE**.

Aubrey

I am not sure when Grandma Judy or Aunt Rhoni joined us but I was so comforted having them with me, with us. Everyone was quiet, listening to the doctors explain that Mom had a pulmonary embolism and they were giving her TPC to break up the blood clots that had invaded her lungs. Then all of a sudden bells started sounding off and I looked over at Mom and it was as if she was gasping for air. Her eyes were open and rolling back in her head. The doctor shouted something at my dad. I don't remember leaving the room.

CODE BLUE was announced yet again and people ran into Mom's room, trying again to save her, to save her for the third time.

Judy

Rhoni and I got there about the same time and the emergency room staff escorted us up to ICU. We were not able to go back until close to 2:30 a.m. The ICU staff were just getting Mary settled into her room. She was unconscious and they had her on life support. Matt, Aubrey, Rhoni, and I were standing at the end of her bed. I was watching the doctors and nurses make sure all the tubes were in place and taking vitals. The doctor explained Mary had a pulmonary embolism. They had administered TPC which is a highly toxic blood clot buster and they were hopeful.

I saw Mary open her eyes. My first response was excitement. Then she opened her mouth and was gasping, although she had a breathing tube. All of it was very odd. Alarms started going off and Mary was dying in front of all of us. The doctor jumped astride her and asked Matt if it was okay to resuscitate. The four of us were escorted out of her room into the hallway where we could still watch what was happening, but we just collapsed on the floor under her window. **CODE BLUE** was announced over the intercom. Crying. My son did not want to be a widower at such a young age. Knowing Mary, she would do everything to stay alive.

Pastor Rick was there. We had a good talk and laugh about my sweet Mary. Her cooking skills stories were a point of much-needed distraction. Minutes ticked by. The longer they were trying to save her, the more worried Matt became. We all were.

Fifteen minutes later the doctor asked Matt to step into Mary's room. I did not want to leave him alone. No matter what the outcome, I knew he needed me.

Rhoni

I have never seen someone die before. It was a pretty violent act of saving someone—it was horrifying. When we were escorted out of Mary's room and **CODE BLUE** was announced over the intercom system, I was holding Aubrey as we were on the floor outside of Mary's room. Everyone was scared and crying and Aubrey asked me if it was wrong to have hope. I didn't know what to say. I felt like this might be the end of her life, but I knew I needed to answer my niece. So I told her that it is never wrong to have hope.

Aubrey

It was just too much. Too much to witness, too many thoughts. I crashed against the wall outside of her room. Aunt Rhoni sat down next to me and held me and we cried. Just cried. I asked my aunt if it was wrong, if it was selfish, to have hope. Through her own tears, she said, "It's never wrong to hope."

I wanted to tell Mom I loved her. I wanted to laugh at her ridiculous jokes. I wanted….I wanted...I wanted.

Dad and Grandma joined us on the floor; I was scared for Dad. I have never seen him cry like that. A desperate plea. No one could talk. We just held on.

Pastor Rick, the hospital chaplain, came over and knelt down with us. He has never met Mom or any of us for that matter. He was quiet. Then simply said, "Tell me something about Mary." I don't remember what anyone said or if they shared loving thoughts or stories or if they just sat there holding onto each other. But I blurted out, "She's a horrible cook!" Dad gently squeezed my hand.

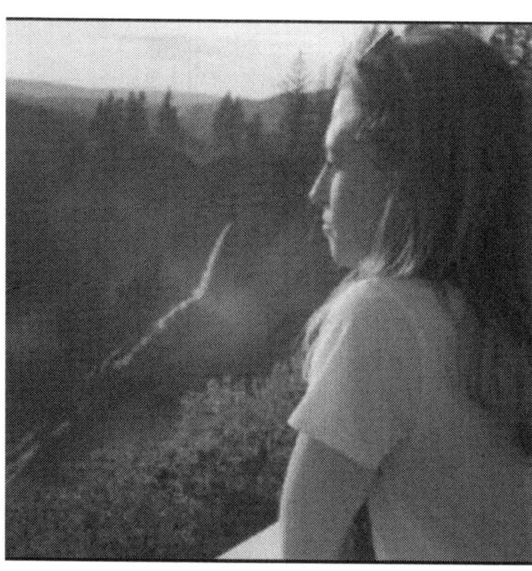

Aubrey

Yup, I want you all to know the very worse quality of Mom is she's a disaster in the kitchen. I mean it. She once burnt toast and placed the toaster outside overnight. So, the next morning she was optimistic and retrieved the toaster from the front stoop. Determination she was not short on. She plugged in the toaster, placed frozen waffles inside, and pushed the lever down. No big deal, right? She turned her head to make a cup of coffee and earwigs started scattering from the toaster. She screamed; smoke was coming from the toaster...well not smoke, but scorched earwigs. She quickly unplugged the toaster and tossed, nope, threw the thing in the yard. She ran back inside and was trying diligently to catch all the earwigs that escaped the firing incinerator only to have their lives taken by a mad woman screaming "Earwigs, earwigs!" All Emily and I could do was laugh!

Mom is such a bad cook she even has a hard time boiling water. Honestly. When we first moved to Colorado she was going to boil eggs, but the water wouldn't boil. She placed eggs in the water thinking something was wrong with the stove. Fifteen minutes later we here explosive sounds coming from the kitchen. The eggs exploded! They were everywhere! Oh, Mom! You are a disaster in the kitchen but it's a charming quality!

These stories are not what I was going to share with Pastor Rick. For some reason, I took it upon myself to ask for forgiveness for Mom's cunningness to fool everyone.

Grandma and Rhoni came to Mom's defense right away. I think it was in unison. "She's not anymore, she made a delicious Thanksgiving Dinner last year."

Through broken breath and tears, I screamed, "It was a premade dinner from Costco!"

Yup, Mom was on her deathbed, fighting for her life, and I outed her on our family secret!

Time. Time is a precious gift never to be taken lightly. Five minutes passed, then ten. The hospital staff didn't stop fighting for her. No one was giving up, so I wouldn't either.

Not only was I feeling guilty for my selfish attitude the past few days, but I was also feeling guilty for telling them her secret. I felt like the worst person ever. I just needed her, I wanted her to forgive me.

Dad was asked to speak privately by one of the doctors. Grandma went with him, knowing he would need support. Planning for the worst, hoping for the best. God had another plan!

Judy

We went back into Mary's room. She was tied down. She had begun swelling and her vitals were stable although weak. The hecticness of the hospital staff had subsided and the doctor explained that Mary was most likely brain-dead. Her pupils were blown out which is indicative of brain death. All we could do is continue to talk to her. He did talk to Matt about making a decision now, in case she were to code again, about continuing with the life-saving efforts or letting her go peacefully. He grabbed Matt's shoulder and said, "No decision has to be made now. Talk to Mary."

I stayed with my son as long as he wanted me to. He pulled up a chair alongside her bed, gently held her hand, which was tied down, and cried. I did not know how to comfort him or what to say. I knew he needed me but I didn't really know what to do. So I closed my eyes and prayed.

Matt

My thoughts went like this: *They don't know MY Mary! They don't know her fight! The news from the doctors didn't hold much hope. They told me to start preparing mentally for what to do if she were to code again. But I believe in her! I believe in us!*

David and Carla

We arrived early on the morning of November 22. When we landed I had tried calling Matt, but it went directly to voicemail. I then called Aubrey. Once again, directly to voicemail. Carla and I had a short wait to get a rental car, then we made the quick drive to the hospital.

When we arrived we went to the emergency room. They would not give us any information at first, but thank goodness there is still human decency. One of the staff nurses must have sensed our urgency and told us they had moved her to ICU.

Carla and I arrived in the ICU. The staff was being very guarded about Mary. They sent for Judy Murphy who met us in the lobby. Judy shared with us that Mary had a pulmonary embolism. She coded three times and it was not good; the doctors were not giving us much hope. She tried to prepare us for seeing Mary on life support. She was trying to be delicate but we could see the worry.

When we were allowed to see Mary, she was in critical condition. Machines were keeping her alive. She did not look like my spunky sister, nor did she look at peace. My heart was hurting terribly to see Matt broken, holding her hand, and Aubrey on the other side of her massaging her other hand, unable to see through the tears. Rhoni stepped outside to take a phone call. It was her dad, letting her know to expect them in the morning and asking for updates.

Carla walked over to Matt and gently touched his shoulder to let him know he was not alone. When he looked up to see us the pain was tangible, the gut-wrenching heartache.

Mary's neurologist came into the room and asked to speak with Matt. Heavy-hearted, he stood up and asked me to join him. The two of us stepped outside her room, neither wanting to leave. Carla took Matt's seat and spoke so lovingly to Mary. I did everything I could not to be emotional but was failing terribly. I pulled myself together, determined I was going to help Matt help Mary.

The doctor told us that things had not changed. She was still in critical condition. There were no signs of brain activity. He was trying to prepare us for the grim reality that she was not with us any longer. He explained they would keep her on life support as long as needed, but we should begin preparing for the final goodbye. Matt was broken. I began asking questions. One was "Is there any hope, any hope at all, that she can pull through?" I pleaded with the doctor to say something, anything, to give us a glimmer of hope.

He then shared he has seen patients with similar conditions pull through and walk out of the hospital. That's all we needed at that time. Whether or not it was true, it's what we needed, what Matt needed. Matt made his way back into Mary's room. Heavy footsteps, heavy-hearted. Just then, Dan called, so I stepped in the waiting room alone so we could talk.

Dan

I called David, who was already with Matt and Mary. He shared that Mary was in ICU and had coded a third time. It was not good and it was best for us both to be there as soon as we could. David spoke very plainly and pointedly, "Dan, Mary might not make it. Mom needs to be here. You need to be here. It's not good." Just then, David broke down crying and said, "I can't be the strong one right now! I can't be Mary's hero. I can't fix this." I assured David that we would do everything possible to get there.

David

As I made my way back to Mary's room I began looking around the surroundings. I noticed how diligent the staff was. Everything that had to be done was being done. Carla was with Matt and Aubrey, doing what she does best: loving, caring, and sitting in silence. Just being. I prayed, for the first time in such a long time. I prayed.

CHAPTER 6

Broken Hallelujah

Me

I hope I never forget what I am going to tell you next. Matt believes from what I can describe that I was in ICU and had already coded three times.

My memory of that time:

I remember feeling at peace.

I was watching someone straddle me and give me chest compressions. My body was flailing like a floppy fish trying to breathe air when it's not supposed to be out of water. Doctors and nurses were running in and out of my room. Commands were being shouted although I could not hear anything. I only remember seeing the hurried and worried expressions. The overall excitement and hecticness of what was happening to my shell—my body that gave birth to two beautiful creations, that loved and celebrated, wept and mourned, was only a shell. I was still alive just in a different form.

As I was watching all of this happen, a bright light appeared from the corner of the room. The light was pure. It did not burn me but was warm, magnificent, comforting, and inviting. I didn't see his face or the color of his skin but his arms opened up and next thing I know HE is holding me close and I rested my head on His chest.

I truly believe with everything in me, that HE was Jesus. I share this with you hesitantly because HE never introduced Himself. I just knew in my heart it was whom I believe was Jesus. I was home! I was safe! I was loved and at peace! Peace is what I felt at the time, perfect peace in every way. No pain. No fear. No confusion. Just peace.

As HE was holding me, cradled in his arms, He told me, "You must go back now."

I was so hurt. I didn't want to go back. I wanted to be with Him. I cried, "But, I want to be with you." At that time I wasn't thinking about Matt, Aubrey, Emily, or those that I love and who love me. I just knew I wanted to be with Jesus.

Jesus then kissed me on my forehead and tells me HE is and always will be with me. He said, "Your job is not done and you must go back."

Now understand, I did simple math for a living. I was confused.

Then suddenly, my dad's silhouette appeared and yelled at me, "Get the hell back there now!" (Dad left us on December 17, 1992.)

Wait, where was I? Could you use that word here in front of Jesus?

As I was being held and feeling loved not wanting to leave, not wanting to go back to my life, not wanting to be the wife to Matt and mother to our two beautiful, caring daughters, I saw the silhouette of my mother-in-law's husband, Phil. He said in his whimsical way, "Tell Judy I love her." (Phil had just passed away September 11, 2013.)

I don't remember going back into my body.

My next memory is on December 3, 2013, waking up to Matt singing our song to me as tears of hope streamed down his gentle face.

CHAPTER 7

Prayers and Miracles

November 22, 2013 (continued)

Rhoni

Early in the morning of November 22, I drove to Denver to pick up my niece Emily. Trying hard to be factual and hopeful, I was preparing Emily for what Mary would look like in ICU, and give her the latest update from the doctors.

I was able to provide some comfort with sharing that her Uncle David and Aunt Carla made their emergency flight and arrived around 4 a.m. I had explained that her Dad was not alone, Grandma Judy was staying close by in case he needed her, and Uncle David and Aunt Carla were caring for Aubrey. I was hoping this would provide some comfort for her. But the tears were heavy.

I told her that Grandpa Ron and Grandma June were almost here and Grandma Karen and her Uncle Dan were on their way. I tried desperately to help but all Em could do was let the tears of fear fall from her brilliant blue eyes. Mary's eyes.

David

Carla and I took Aubrey to the cafeteria for breakfast around 8 a.m. Matt stayed in the room holding Mary's hand and reading to her all of the beautiful messages and prayers that were being sent.

Judy

Around 8 a.m., I was watching Matt and Mary. I stood outside her room peering through the large window the nurses use to monitor every movement. No one had hope. I had overheard the staff talking about my Mary, expecting another cardiac arrest. Even though her vitals were stable, she was still unresponsive, and her eyes still dilated. I didn't want to leave, but I didn't want to be in the way. I desperately prayed for God to give her another chance. My son was brave as he held onto her hand gently caressing it and whispering through heavy tears. David and Carla took Aubrey down to the cafeteria for breakfast and Rhoni left to get Emily from Denver.

It had been a very long night. Matt would not leave Mary's side. He said, "In case she were to wake up I didn't want her to be alone." Hope. He had an abundance of hope.

Matt's Blog: Mary Kaye's Odyssey

Friday, November 22, 2013

Posted November 23, 2013, 1:16 p.m. by Matthew Podschweit. [Updated December 1, 2013, 12:10 p.m.]

We have Mary Kaye in a room in the ICU and my sister Rhoni and my mom Judy arrive. We are in the room with MK discussing the events so far, when suddenly alarms start sounding and MK is crashing for a third time. The attending physician jumps astride MK on the bed and begins chest compressions. I've never actually seen this done in person before, and I am shocked at how utterly violent it is. Doctors and nurses are buzzing like bees in and out, and as the four of us retreat into the hallway, a Code Blue is announced over the PA. We are emotionally distraught—Aubrey will recount that she has never seen me cry so hard. Through the blur of the events, we find ourselves crouched in the hallway, balled up in a group hug on the floor. The activity in MK's room slowly begins to calm down, and the specialist comes out to talk to us. He explains that MK is on life support—machines breathing for her, drugs are keeping her heart beating and blood pressure at safe levels. He says that neurological damage is likely, and that they can sustain life support indefinitely, but that this may be as good as it gets.

So we wait. As we get into the wee hours of the morning, the nurses begin trying to stir a response from MK by speaking loudly to her as they attend to her machines and tubes and wires. There is the occasional flutter of her eyelids, but no sign of waking. Soon we notice that MK has partially opened her eyes, but is still unresponsive. Her arms and legs are moving slightly, stirring as if trying to find a comfortable position. A while later (I have absolutely NO recollection of how long) she opens her eyes and appears to be awake. She appears very confused and is scanning the room with her eyes, but when one of the nurses calls her name, she looks right at her. This is totally unexpected. As we continue to hold her hands and evoke a response from MK, we can feel slight squeezes, and when we ask her to squeeze, she does.

The nurses tell us they have never seen anyone in MK's condition progress so rapidly. It is not long before she attempts to communicate with us. We explain to MK that she can't talk because she has a tube in her mouth, and I feel her hand moving in mine. She is signing something, spelling a word. I asked her to start over, and she signs "W" and then "A," and then...I don't recognize the letter. I asked her to repeat it, which she does, but of course, I'm not going to recognize it simply because she does it again (duh!). So I start with "A" and she shakes her head slightly. "B"? Another shake, and so on, until "T"—a nod.

"WAT" and she makes an "E"—she wants water! My heart almost jumps out of my chest! Unfortunately, she can't have any water—it would go straight down her windpipe because of the tubes, but she's aware enough to spell a word to me in sign language. I cannot adequately express how encouraged I am at this point. Prayers and miracles will be the theme of this day forever!

Emily

When I landed in Denver after a long and lonely trip from Miami I was so grateful to see my Aunt Rhoni. I asked her to fill me in. She shared with me, tried to prepare me, but nothing could have helped. I was distraught.

Rhoni and I arrived at St. Francis Hospital in Colorado Springs around 9 a.m. I sprinted to the ICU. When I got there, Dad, Aubrey, Grandma Judy, Uncle David, and Aunt Carla were waiting for me and Aunt Rhoni to join them. I was winded from sprinting to ICU. They explained that Grandma Karen, Uncle Dan, Grandpa Ron, and Grandma June were on their way. Grandma Karen and Uncle Dan were caught in an ice storm but were on standby and Grandpa Ron and Grandma June were flying out today. They also tried to prepare me for what Mom was going to look like.

Dad held me gently in his arms. He shared Mom was on life support. She was swollen and did not look like herself. The doctors had first explained that she was most likely brain-dead but she was showing signs of consciousness. That's all we needed at that time. Hope! Dad would never let go of hope.

Dad and I walked to her room in ICU. I remember looking through the glass window in disbelief at what I was seeing. She didn't look like my mom. I was not going to go in. I saw Dad go into the room and take this woman's hand and lovingly hold it. I ran out of ICU, frantic, in disbelief. Aubrey held me as I sobbed. Grandma Judy said, "Sweetie, it's important she knows you are here. Go talk to her." Grandma walked me to the door of ICU. I stood in the doorway. She didn't look like Mom but I knew it was her, it had to be. She was so, well, so huge. Her kidneys and heart were failing. She was on life-saving machines, in and out of consciousness.

I stepped into the room. Tears ran down my face; my eyes were blurry with fright. Dad didn't know I was in the room. I watched and listened as my dad read to her through blurry eyes all the loving messages people had been sending and then said, "Honey, Emily is on her way here. She will want to see that beautiful smile of yours."

I touched his shoulder very gently and said, “Dad, I’m right here."

We burst into tears. Dad got up and once again held me. "You are such a strong, brave girl," he whispered, with a brokenness I was not expecting.

The doctor came in and asked to speak to him. So he stepped just outside the door. I was left alone with Mom. I sat down next to her where Dad was just sitting. Not knowing what to say or how to speak over the sounds of the ventilator and all the monitors. I start rubbing her arm as the disbelief was quickly turning into reality. Then anger came over me. I said, “Mom, why didn’t you listen? Why didn’t you go to the hospital when I said it sounds like a blood clot? You cannot leave us, do you understand, fight for Dad, fight for us...I don’t care what it takes, just fight!”

Mom opened her eyes, looked so dazed and confused. I said, “There you are!” and just like that she closed them.

Uncle David and Aunt Carla joined Dad outside the room with the doctors. Perfect timing. Dad was not alone. It was always better to have additional input and questions that can be asked. Dad was doing the best he could.

"Good news," Dad said, "They are going to remove the intubation tube tomorrow morning."

Ron and June (Matt's dad and stepmom)

We made our way directly to the hospital late in the morning of November 22. Once we arrived in the ICU waiting room Matt, Emily, and Judy were with Mary. David and Carla had flown in from Arizona and were caring for Aubrey. Rhoni was filling us in on all that had occurred since we last spoke.

Once Aubrey saw us she came over and held me, her grandpa, and cried, something I will cherish for all of my days. David shared that Karen and Dan were on standby to fly out during a break in the ice storm and would be here on the next available flight.

CHAPTER 8

Hope in a Smile

November 23, 2013

Dan

Dave kept us informed of everything that was going on. At times it looked hopeful but other times not. I kept our conversations private. I wasn't sure Mom could handle the rollercoaster of ups and downs. Our flight landed in Denver and Shelly, my amazing wife, had made arrangements for our rental car and hotel ahead of time so we could go directly to the hospital.

Matt's Blog: Mary Kaye's Odyssey

Saturday, November 23, 2013

Posted November 23, 2013, 3:49 p.m. by Matthew Podschweit. [Updated December 1, 2013, 12:09 p.m.]

Dave and Carla Decker relieved me at 8 p.m. Friday night and the girls and I went home to get some rest. After rearranging the furniture that was rather haphazardly placed by the paramedics during MK's triage, I put on my

PJs, cracked a beer, and joined the girls in the basement for some light NetFlix'n. It didn't take long for the fatigue to set in, and I was out like a light by 10:30. The girls got some sleep and then relieved Dave and Carla at about midnight, and I returned to the hospital this morning about 8 a.m. MK had been off the blood pressure medicine and the epinephrine for a while, and since she was maintaining a good blood pressure on her own, the nurse gave her a mild sedative so she would rest more comfortably. I took the girls down to the cafeteria and got them breakfast, and sent them home to clean the house and go to bed (in that order!). As I sat with MK, she awoke, looked at me and, as best as she could, mouthed the question "What happened?" I briefly told her, and then she slowly closed her eyes and dozed off for a while. This sequence of events repeated itself several times. My good friend Jon shared with me that this happened to him when he suffered complete cardiac arrest several years ago. He recounts that he was technically dead for ten minutes and was revived. Although he has no memory of the few days that followed, he was told that he would repeat the same question about every thirty seconds, as if his brain was restarting over and over. Aside from Jon being one of my favorite people in the world, his story gives me great hope and encouragement!

I can't help but be excited because Uni, MK's daytime nurse, said sometime this afternoon MK's breathing tube will come out. She needs to rest, relax, and breathe slowly and deeply, so Uni has mandated no visitors until MK sees the doctor. Our family and friends have constructed a refugee camp in the lobby, circling the chairs like Conestoga Wagons and fashioning makeshift beds for quick naps. MK's brother Dan and my mom Karen are arriving today, and just as we were hoping, MK's breathing tube came out just before they made their appearance. We all wanted to spare Karen the shock of seeing MK with that big tube in her mouth, even though Karen's former profession was a registered nurse—I'm sure she's seen far worse than that. Uni came out just as Karen and Dan were getting off the elevator. She said she would let ALL of us come down to see MK for just a couple of minutes, and then MK would need to rest and concentrate on her breathing.

We marched in formation around Karen's wheelchair down the hall to MK's room, and then filed in and formed a semicircle around the foot of her bed. I walked in last, just in time to see MK whisper the word "WOW" and then I saw something I thought I might never see again—MK's smile! I could not contain the joy bursting from my heart, and tears ran like rain down my face. I don't know how long we will be on this road, but if I can still count on MK's smile, we will weather whatever lies ahead!

Karen (Mary's mom)

We arrived in Colorado Springs the day of November 23. When Dan and I arrived the family was waiting for us as we got off the elevator. They shared with us that Mary was responding, so they were in the process of removing the breathing tube. Matt was asked to step out of the room while they did thc procedure. He had a hard time not being next to her but the nurses explained they would come and get him as soon as they could. He was relieved to have all of us together. Mary would have loved being there.

The nurse came out and said we could all go in together. All of us! She said we could only be with her for a few minutes but it was a few minutes of much needed time.

We all went into her ICU room together. Matt, Aubrey, Emily, David, Carla, Rhoni and her husband, David and their two girls, Alex and Kennedy, Judy, Ron, June, and finally me and Dan. All of us had made the trip. Dan rolled me in first and I couldn't stop crying. After all she had been through, she smiled! My heart exploded with love and gratitude towards God. She smiled and then closed her eyes. The monitors were sounding off in the typical pattern of life. For now, she was fighting. For now, she was with us.

We were allowed only ten minutes to be with her. Then the doctors came in and said they needed to speak with Matt and asked that everyone else wait outside. Matt asked if I could stay in the room and the doctor was hesitant but said yes. Matt invited David and Danny to join him. I am certain he was exhausted and overwhelmed. His love for my Mary has always been obvious but now it was more evident. He wanted to do right by her and knew he needed some help with decisions.

I was left alone with my little girl for some much needed and very precious time. Dan had wheeled my chair next to the window and Mary Kaye's left hand. The marks on her wrist from being tied down were turning into bruises. She was in and out of consciousness. Her heart rate was becoming very erratic. I was so afraid, so scared for her, Matt, Aubrey, and Emily. I always thought Mary was a wonderful wife and mother, and for our family not to have her in our lives was too much. I wanted her to wake up, to tell me she was here and that she loved me.

I could hear the nurses talk about my girl and the outlook was very grim. They were preparing for Mary to code a fourth time. A nurse came over and asked if she could wheel me to the waiting room. Mary's vitals were not good. Her monitors were giving off warning signals. My eyes flooded with tears. I asked if I could just have a few minutes. She simply gave me a warm smile and nodded yes.

I grabbed her hand, and said, "Honey, do you remember the song we would sing together? It was your favorite song and you would curl up on my lap and say, "'Sing it again, Mama.'" Truly hoping for some recognition or response, I would have taken anything at that moment, but her heart rate was too fast, and her breathing too shallow.

I began singing to her as I held her hand in mine:

"You are my sunshine, my only sunshine; You make me happy when skies are gray; You'll never know dear, how much I love you. Please don't take my sunshine away."

I couldn't hold down the tears as they cascaded down my face. My voice quivered as I sang. The nurses gathered at the door and witnessed our love as her heart rate stabilized. Glory be to God!

Dan

We arrived. Everyone was waiting for us in the lobby. The staff was removing her breathing tube. I saw Matt, he looked exhausted, overwhelmed and grateful. All the hellos were not even done and the updates were not finished when Mary's nurse came out and shared that we could all go see her. ALL of us! Aubrey and Emily came over and held Mom or Mom held them. Isn't it one and the same?

She did not look like my sister. There were tubes everywhere, and monitors were beeping. My thought was *"I don't want to remember her like this—this is not my sister."* Then she opened her eyes, mouthed "WOW!" and smiled. She smiled, and that was it, she closed her eyes.

A few minutes later the doctor came in and asked to speak to Matt. He asked Dave and me to join him. He didn't have to do this but he knew we would want to, or he needed us to be with him. Either way, I was thankful to be part of this conversation. I just wasn't expecting the news he was about to give. While he escorted us into his office a nurse was beginning to escort everyone out of the room. Matt turned around and asked if Mom could stay with her. When the doctor said yes, I rolled Mom by the window on Mary's left side.

Emotions were running high. The doctor explained that the signs indicated that she had a very high chance of coding again. He reminded Matt of the conversation a few nights ago, after the third time she coded, to prepare to make a decision of continuing to keep her alive or let her go peacefully.

All Matt could say is, "You don't know my Mary. You have to understand that I believe she is fighting to stay."

Dave started asking medical questions about brain damage and quality of life, looking for some reassurance. I couldn't take it so I walked out of the room only to see the nursing staff gathered around Mary's room. Some were crying. My initial thought was "*Oh no, she's gone*." When I walked over to her room I witnessed Mom holding her hand and singing! Her vitals were good!

Mary's nurse said they witnessed another miracle from my sister's fight.

Aubrey

I was holding Mom's hand and telling her stories. Mom always said that I had great empathy, but I had not shown that much lately. I hoped that I could be more for her in the days to come.

Dad was trying to take care of everything else and was making a list of family to be by Mom's side at all times. He was working with the insurance company, communicating with Mom's work, his work, and all of our friends who congregated at the hospital ICU waiting room just to be with our family.

David and Carla

Carla insisted that Matt go home and get some much-needed rest. She and I would be with Mary in case she woke up. He agreed. Judy, Rhoni, and her family all left as well. Our desperation turned into hope. Dan and Mom went to the hotel. Ron and June were staying close by just in case. No one wanted to leave but everyone knew the importance of rest. It was going to be a very long journey and while Matt had the help right now, this was the time for him to rest, to sleep.

Matt insisted that Mary not be alone. He made a schedule for each of us to take a time to be with her. We took the first shift. Mary's vitals were stable now. Carla would read to her while holding her hand, and I would pace.

Aubrey and Emily came to relieve us at midnight. We all wanted Mary to wake up but when she did open her eyes she was scared. She did this frequently. Unable to communicate, uneasy from having to be tied down so she would stop thrashing, she would try to move. She looked so confused and would repeat herself with a struggling voice, "Wow, you look great; what are you doing here?" We would tell her that she is in ICU and it's going to be okay. Her eyes would close and she would thrash all over again. Five minutes later she would open her eyes and look incredibly confused and once again muster, "Wow, you look great; what are you doing here?" and again we would tell her, "You are in ICU and it's going to be okay." This process would be repeated for days.

I didn't want to leave her, but I knew we had to be strong for Matt and we also needed our rest.

Aubrey and Emily

We have just been through forty-eight hours of intense emotion. When we came to the ICU to relieve Uncle David and Aunt Carla, Mom was very agitated. It was scary to see her like that. It wasn't until we would touch her and speak to her that she was able to relax some. We found that rubbing her arm gently helped.

CHAPTER 9

Glimmers of Hope

November 24, 2013

Dave and Carla

When we met Matt in the ICU lobby, he was hopeful, so thankful that Mary had a chance. He knew she was fighting to be with him. He explained that the process with her memory had not improved but she was happy. When we were allowed to go into her room she was sitting up beaming with joy! "David and Carla, it's so nice to see you; what are you doing here?" and then she would close her eyes. About five minutes later, still sitting up, she would see us and once again beam with joy! "David and Carla, it's so nice to you; what are you doing here?" Carla said it must feel like Christmas morning, waking up with joy every five minutes.

Matt's Blog: Mary Kaye's Odyssey

Sunday, November 24, 2013

Posted November 24, 2013, 5:54 p.m. by Matthew Podschweit. [Updated December 1, 2013, 12:07 p.m.]

I have been spared the duty of overnight vigil yet again—Dave and Carla stayed with MK from 8 until midnight, and Aubrey, Emily, and our friend Madison pulled the night shift (youth is quite wasted on the young). MK had a rather restless night I'm told, but managed to get some rest. I arrived back at the hospital about 8:30 a.m. and was greeted by MK's beaming smile. She has been running a slowly descending temperature, and I was relieved to see she had finally broken 100. Shortly after I arrived, her respiratory doctor came in to check on her. He is the doctor that removed the breathing tube yesterday. She had been taking ice chips through the night to relieve her rather sore throat, and perhaps had a few too many. The water upset her stomach and she got a little sick, but no big deal. He asked her a few questions about how she was feeling, and based on the information he collected, determined that they would move her into a regular hospital bed out of ICU tomorrow. Great progress! A little while later, the nurse came in and asked MK if she'd like to get out of bed and sit up in a chair. MK seemed to think for a moment, and then said yes. I think she was surprised by how much effort it took to swing her legs over the side of the bed and sit up, and she took a few minutes to catch her breath before she tried to stand up. Two nurses flanked her as she slowly rose to her feet and turned to sit in the recliner next to her bed. Once we got her pillows situated, she was quite comfortable and I think glad to be vertical.

Her voice is starting to come back, still a little raspy, but much better than yesterday. Her face is showing more expression as she greets family coming in to visit her. She is still a bit confused, and her short-term memory, although getting better, is still keeping her from remembering what happened and where she is. This is normal and to be expected, but there is no denying that she is still MK—gentle, bright, smiling MK, so thankful for the incredible outpouring of love from friends and family all over the country!

I sat next to her and read just the names of all the people who had been texting their well-wishes and prayers, and after that, let her know of the 600+ men's prayer group in an unknown church in Washington that prayed for her, the church in Ft. Lauderdale FL that is praying because I happened to sit next to one of the members on a flight a year ago and stumbled across his number, and of course the incredible church family we have in the Quad Cities! Now that I think about it, how could I expect anything less than a miracle?

Dan

When we walked into Mary's room, she was actually sitting up in a chair! We were so astonished by her progress and she was very happy to see us! She even called me by my name, "*brother Dan*." As we visited it became apparent that she getting uncomfortable and her blood pressure was dropping. The nurses respectfully asked us to leave so that she could rest. Mom kissed her gently on the cheek and told her that we would be back.

CHAPTER 10

Birthday Blessings

Matt's Blog: Mary Kaye's Odyssey

Monday, November 25, 2013

Posted November 26, 2013, 12:44 p.m. by Matthew Podschweit. [Updated December 1, 2013, 12:06 p.m.]

Today starts at 6 a.m. waking up in the lobby. Long night, the wind was blowing like crazy. I didn't get much sleep as I was trying to fit on a way-too-small couch, but I did sleep a little. Time of day is way different for MK right now, so I have no hesitation about coming in to see how she's doing. She's awake and alert, still very confused and asking, "What happened?" and, "Where am I?" but she's happy to see me and I don't mind repeating the story. The nurse comes in and asks MK if she feels like getting up and into a chair this morning. She says sure, and we start to rearrange her tubes and wires. She's very weak but manages to stand and scoot over to the recliner next to the bed. A few deep breaths, the nausea subsides, and she settles in. Kamie (she's the nurse) asks if she'd like to take her breakfast while she's in the chair. They bring her chicken broth, coffee, apple juice, jello, and a popsicle. MK immediately goes for the popsicle! I think her throat is still sore from the breathing tube. She eats most of the popsicle and a sip of juice and she's done.

She is having more pain in her chest and abdomen, and she seems very preoccupied with it. Kamie has been giving her pain medication and is doing so more frequently. We look at MK's monitor and her blood pressure is quite high. I ask and Kamie explains that her pain level will affect her BP that way.

MK's brother Dan and my mom join us. MK is so happy to see them and smiles, but it is apparent that she is quite tired. We visit for a while, and we notice that her BP has climbed to 193/114, very alarming. I notice that MK seems very confused, and she stops responding to my comments and questions. I ask her if she would like to get back in bed and she gives a slight nod and closes her eyes.

This feels like a setback to me. The staff is also concerned about her increasing pain, and Dr. Workman has ordered a CT scan for her abdomen, chest, and head. The scan shows a hematoma next to her spleen that is slowly leaking blood into her abdomen. This is not necessarily dangerous, but because she is currently on blood thinners, they will keep a very close eye on it. Her chest scan is clear and her head scan shows nothing (even MK chuckled a bit when I reported this).

I realized that I forgot to take my migraine pill last night and know that if I skip a dose, I will become "grumpy Daddy" before the end of the day. Emily comes to relieve me at about 11:30 a.m., Aubrey is going to work the lunch shift at P.F. Changs, and Dad, June, Rhoni, Dave, Alex, and Kennedy are all holding vigil in the waiting room. I head home to make some phone calls, answer some emails, take a shower, and keep the laundry going. Returning to the hospital at around 5 p.m., I find MK is quite tired and sleepy. She's going to get a surgical consult regarding the bleeding in her abdomen, but we don't know exactly when. We decide everyone needs a decent meal, so I make sure the nurses have my phone number and we go to The Rock Bottom Restaurant for some food. Just as we are walking in, my phone rings. It's Dr. McCann, her surgical consult. He explains that they are going to perform a procedure tomorrow to place a tiny filter in the main vein leading from her lower body to her torso (vena cava, I believe). He explains that they want to take her off of the blood thinner to speed healing of the hematoma and bruising around her rib cage (this was the result of chest compressions during CPR). The filter is a precaution against clots forming and traveling to her lungs and heart. He is very confident that this will go very smoothly and I find him very reassuring. Back to the hospital after dinner, a kiss goodnight, and Aubrey and Emily are setting up camp in the waiting room.

David

I came to be with Mary while everyone else went out to lunch together. It's our birthday! Yes, Mary and I share the same birthday but six years apart! Carla let me spend some much needed time alone with her. After lunch, Matt came back to the hospital and the girls went home to rest.

Judy, Rhoni, Dave, Alex, and Kennedy all went home up north for the day, after bringing Mary gifts and teasing about how she can open them when she's ready!

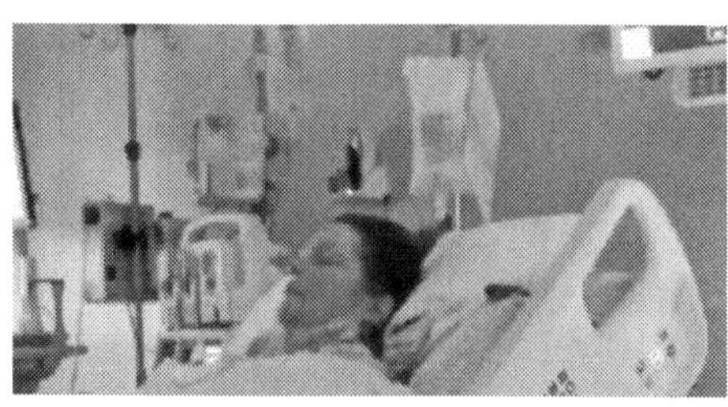

I was glad that Ron and June were staying with Matt. I hoped he was getting rest. I now felt confident that she, my sister, was going to make it. I was a witness to many miracles in Mary's health! I don't know how else to explain everything that she has been through without exploring faith.

My wife is a beautiful person, full of compassion and empathy. When things looked so dark, I would see her with Mary rubbing her arm, telling her stories. I couldn't wait to share these moments with Mary when she was more alert.

Mom, Dan, Carla, and I would head back to our respective homes the next day. Matt assured us he would keep us in the know. Our hope was that she would be moved out of ICU soon and home the next week.

Matt's Blog: Mary Kaye's Odyssey

Tuesday, November 26, 2013

Posted November 26, 2013, 1:51 p.m. by Matthew Podschweit. [Updated December 1, 2013, 12:05 p.m.]

Completely forgot to mention that yesterday was MK's birthday! We have collected several gifts for her, but we're waiting for a time when MK is better able to enjoy a little party. I arrive at the hospital at about 8:40 a.m. to find Aubrey in the waiting room, sleeping on a couch. Emily must be in MK's room. I have chai tea for Em, caramel macchiato for Aubrey, fruit and muffins, and my venti Americano with room for cream (as usual). My friends from Heritage will not be surprised that Jenn Swift and the Hamptons very lovingly delivered Coke and Snickers bars a few days ago, but I barely got access to them as the girls seem to have acquired Dad's affinity for this junky combination.

I walk into MK's room to her lovely, beaming smile. Emily says she's been asking for me and she's glad I'm here. MK's blood pressure is much better, about 138/89 and her temp is normal. Dr. Williams, Dr. Workman, Carrie the speech pathologist, Marva the caseworker, and then Chris the cath lab tech make rounds through the room, and then it's off to her procedure. Dr. VanWagenen (spelling is a total guess, but the idea that he's probably Belgian is not) is doing the procedure. I sign the release and head to the ICU waiting room. This should take about a half hour, and right on cue, Dr. VanWagenen comes out to let us know everything went well. MK will spend a couple hours in her ICU room, and then we will follow her ambulance across town to Penrose Hospital where a regular hospital room awaits her.

Just heard from Dr. Williams—Penrose, the main campus facility and where they were going to send MK this afternoon, is full. Therefore, she is going to stay put in ICU at St. Francis for the next couple of days.

OK, scratch that. The hematoma next to MK's spleen is slowly leaking blood into her abdominal cavity. I'm told that this is only a minor complication; the bleeding should stop and the body will simply absorb the blood over time. The problem is blood collecting where it doesn't belong causes a great deal of pressure which causes a lot of pain. Amanda, MK's nighttime nurse, has been working very hard trying to get MK transferred over to Penrose because, as the main campus, they have more resources than St. Francis—surgeons and radiologists on site around the clock, advanced machinery, and a larger ICU. Amanda does not anticipate MK will need surgery but would feel better just in case. I get the impression that Amanda is one of those individuals that knows how to make friends, influence people, and get things to happen. By 10:15 p.m. we are loading MK into an ambulance and it's lights and sirens across town to Penrose.

CHAPTER 11

The Curiosity of Kennedy

Matt's Blog: Mary Kaye's Odyssey

Wednesday, November 27, 2013

Posted November 27, 2013, 12:33 p.m. by Matthew Podschweit. [Updated December 1, 2013, 12:04 p.m.]

Settling into our new digs in the Penrose ICU, MK is in a lot of pain. It's really hard to see her like this; I wish there was something more that I could do besides assuring her that everything that could be done is being done and trying to distract her from her discomfort. We try breathing together like we learned during Lamaze classes at Illini hospital in Silvis, IL. This actually seems to be pretty effective, and even brings her blood pressure down a little.

She has been more lucid today and her short-term memory seems to be improving. She's retaining new information better, and is remembering where she is and why she's there. It's a really good sign. But now there is a very tenuous balancing act taking place—pain meds are maxed which makes her loopy and slurs her speech, blood pressure medicine is working against the pain that raises her BP, vitamin K is being administered to reverse the effects of the Coumadin so the vessel in her abdomen will stop hemorrhaging—it's dizzying, really.

Rhoni and Kennedy (my sister and niece, respectively) have come down from Lakewood at about noon to give me a little break. They are sitting with MK while I take Dad and June out and about Colorado Springs. We hit Panera Bread because I've got a hankerin' for Mac 'n Cheese. Diana, my boss, joins us. I haven't seen Di since last Wednesday; she was out of town administrating coaching clinics in Ft. Walton Beach, FL. I would make a sarcastic remark like, "Wow, tough gig," but she had three separate courses running simultaneously, so I know she didn't get any beach time, let alone much time to herself at all.

Dad and June have never been to the office, so after lunch, we head there for a tour. It's the day before Thanksgiving, so chances are many staff will be off, but it's really nice to make the rounds after being off almost a full week. It's hard to keep my composure, there has been such an outpouring of love and kindness from these people (thanks a lot, Barkley—actually I mean that).

It's 4:00 p.m. and I'm feeling I really need to get back to the hospital. We run Emily home and then back downtown, it takes almost an hour. I walk into MK's room to find her visiting with Rhoni and Kennedy. MK smiles when she sees me and I can tell she's feeling better. Not only has the pain lessened a great deal, her blood pressure is a much improved 117/68. Her pain medication is still being delivered at a high rate and dosage, so she is still quite sleepy and her speech is a little slurred, but she's smiling and beautiful and alive!

Kennedy (Rhoni and David's daughter)

I have been taking the time to sit with my Aunt Mary in the ICU, watching the staff be so attentive, and curious about the science behind the medications and the monitors. It was all so fascinating to me! I do not feel afraid.

Aunt Mary was always a jokester and when she smiled at me and her eyes twinkled, I knew she was there! That was all that I needed! I kept waiting for her to tell a joke or do something to make me laugh but I had to wait a little longer for that moment. That is where I have learned great patience!

I had many concerns about my Aunt Mary's care. The doctors and nurses were very kind to indulge me, and answer my curious questions regarding the science behind what they were doing to help her.

CHAPTER 12

The Thanksgiving Toast

Matt's Blog: Mary Kaye's Odyssey

Thursday, November 28, 2013

Posted November 28, 2013, 8:18 p.m. by Matthew Podschweit. [Updated December 1, 2013, 12:04 p.m.]

Happy Thanksgiving. We had a nice day with the family, 10:00 a.m. brunch reservations, early afternoon in the hospital waiting room filing two-by-two in to see MK. We left about 3:30 p.m. and let MK rest while we headed back to our house to watch Dallas vs. Oakland (sorry Jimmy, Raiders can't seem to get a break). Dad and June, Mom, Dave, Rhoni, Alex and Kennedy, Aubrey and Emily—thank you so much for being such a loving, drama-free family.

Everyone has left and it's just me, Aubrey, and Emily sorting through the food, cards, and flowers that have been so kindly contributed to sustain us through this chapter. My phone rings at 5:50 p.m. and I don't recognize the number. It's the hospital, and MK is not feeling well. She's quite anxious and asking for me, so I grab my backpack and head out the door. The girls have decided to pull the night shift again (bless them) and they are just behind me. I arrive and MK is fidgeting uncomfortably. I ask her "Where does it hurt?" to which she replies, "Everywhere." It's an answer, but not very informative. Laura her nurse tells me she's taking MK down for another CT scan to see if something is going on in her belly. They wheel her away and I realize I've left my backpack in the car, so I sign out and go to the car. When I return, it is 6:35 p.m.—nurse shift change, and I'm locked out till 8. Dang.

I've managed to get back to see MK before 8, nurse Laura has called me back at MK's request. The CT scan shows that another hematoma has formed in her abdomen and is filling her abdominal cavity again. There is a suggestion that Interventive Radiology may do a procedure similar to the one that placed the screen in MK's vena cava, but this time find the vessel that's bleeding and coil it off, stopping the bleeding. After a consult, they decide not to do the procedure and MK will just have to gut it out again. The girls have been allowed to join me in MK's room and are now massaging her hands and feet with stress relief eucalyptus lotion and the whole room smells like menthol. Could be worse.

Balancing the medication that thins and coagulates the blood is evidently very complicated and requires a great deal of trial and error. It takes time to evaluate even a slight adjustment, and it's difficult to be patient when someone you love is uncomfortable and waiting for relief. Emily is combing MK's hair and Aubrey is painting her toenails. I'm sitting here typing. I guess we're all keeping busy. This really seems to have calmed MK though, and she has stopped squirming and moaning. Hoping for a quiet night, guess we'll see.

David (Rhoni's husband)

Well, if this wasn't a prank, Mary Kaye was probably laughing at another Thanksgiving joke! Remembering the Costco Thanksgiving meal from the last year—the cat was out of the bag! Thank you, Aubrey! I couldn't wait to tease her about that one!

As we were sitting around for brunch, I decided to toast Mary Kaye and I had the whole restaurant join us in standing and shouting out "*Mary!*" at the same time! I know that she would have loved that moment!

CHAPTER 13

Life in the Extremes

Matt's Blog: Mary Kaye's Odyssey

Friday, November 29, 2013

Posted November 29, 2013, 1:17 p.m. by Matthew Podschweit. [Updated December 1, 2013, 12:03 p.m.]

This morning starts with the sound of the garage door opening at about 6:45 a.m. The girls are home from their overnight shift with MK. "How's your Mom this morning?" I ask through the blur of just-opened eyes. "She got a little crazy last night," Aubrey answers. MK got anxious yesterday with her pain increasing and the confining, claustrophobic feeling of the web of tubes and wires, not to mention being rather bloated from retaining fluid. The nurse gave her some anxiety medicine and that's when the fun began. She has become quite talkative and animated and a little silly. At one point, she called me, "A lovely married-to-me man." I told her that title is too long to put on my business cards, but I appreciated the sentiment. "Do you think Ellen DeGeneres has ever experienced intensive care before? Because I think I sound like Dori, you know, when she's trying to talk to the whale, "Ohhh Kaaaaay!"

MK's vitals look really good—BP is 118/81, 02 saturation is 96% and pulse is 88 bpm. It's noon and I'm ready for some lunch. MK is starting to settle down a little, maybe she'll take a nap and I can run and get some food.

IR is still considering the procedure to coil off the bleeding vessel in her belly, but they will wait until they've tested her blood to see what her red blood cell count is. I'm guessing they will not.

It's 9:10 p.m. and MK's anxiety is proving to be something else. We thought maybe she was having a reaction to the anxiety medication, so we stopped giving it to her, but there was no change. She is experiencing involuntary tics and movements and vocalizations—her behavior and speech is sometimes silly and childlike and bordering on bizarre. She is very uncomfortable and getting loud. We finally get the doctor's attention and he has ordered another CT scan of her head. I'm worried about her and the girls are here at the hospital with me. I will report back once I hear from the doctor.

Aubrey

The medicine they were giving Mom was having a reverse effect. It was making her involuntary muscle movement much worse, even though the idea was for her to get some rest. When the nurse came in to inject her IV with muscle relaxant, Emily began yelling! She told them it was clearly the medicine that was making it worse and they needed to stop! She was a spitfire! Emily wasn't trying to hurt anyone's feelings, but she was concerned about Mom. I tried to calm her and explained that they were doing the best they could. But I could see that Emily could sense that Mom was overmedicated.

The only way to stop Mom from writhing in pain was if someone was massaging either her feet or hands. Physical touch was so important to her being grounded.

Matt's Blog: Mary Kaye's Odyssey

Saturday, November 30, 2013

Posted November 30, 2013, 12:24 p.m. by Matthew Podschweit. [Updated December 1, 2013, 12:02 p.m.]

There is no catharsis in this post. I can't find any comfort in expressing the state of things right now, there is too much up in the air. Please pray for MK. I spoke with Dr. Pennington this morning about 9:15 a.m. They provided MK with enough sedation last night that she has gotten some restful sleep, and for that I am very grateful. When she is awake, she continues to writhe and vocalize mostly unintelligibly, but responds to our requests. She is able to swallow water and pills with some help, but carrying on a conversation is not feasible. She becomes very agitated when people are around, especially me and the girls. It's hard to see her in this state, but harder to leave the room, even knowing that she is much more likely to settle down and rest when we're not there. Please intercede for MK through prayer.

Dr. Pennington believes she is reacting adversely to the sedative medications she's been given, and so they have taken her off all of those. He does not believe this is an adverse reaction to the pain medication they have been giving her. He has scheduled an MRI for this morning, specifically looking for any sign of permanent damage to her brain that may have occurred during the times she coded, but he's fairly confident that we are seeing one of two possible causes—adverse reaction to medication or something called "ICU Psychosis"—anxiety brought about by extended time spent in a critical care environment. First, the MRI, next, observe over the next 24 hours how she responds to being taken off the sedatives and third, evaluate for ICU psychosis.

I am not blind to the spiritual aspects of this situation. Please continue to pray for healing and against any evil that would plot to defile or bring harm to one of Christ's most beautiful living examples of His love. This type of intercession is not a last resort, it is an ongoing battle, fought knowing that in the end, love will win the day.

MK's MRI has come back normal. Praise God! Tomorrow is a brand new day.

Emily

I tried to convince Dad that I should stay and help. He quickly shut that idea down saying, "Mom would want you to go back to school to be around your teammates, coaches and in your classes."

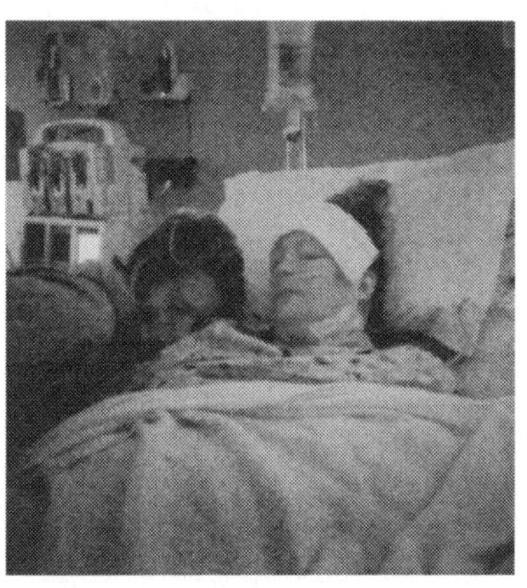

Emily and Mary Kaye

I got a little mad and said, "Dad, it's what I want." He looked at me puzzled. "Em, do you really?" he asked.

Only after a few brief moments I said, "Dad, you are right, I need to go back." My beach coach, mentor and friend, Krissy Bredehoft, had been waiting with my family in lobby of ICU. She volunteered to take me to the Denver airport.

But, first I had to say goodbye to Mom. I was no longer mad at her. I admired her fight. I realized how her love and faith has impacted so many. Friends from everywhere came to just be in the lobby of the hospital. The food, flowers, and cards were overwhelming.

I was overwhelmed with love for my mom, I held her hand as she rested, and kissed her head. Tears filled my eyes as I said, "Goodbye," and then I quietly left to head back to school.

CHAPTER 14

The Doctor and The Rubber Mallet

Matt's Blog: Mary Kaye's Odyssey

Sunday, December 1, 2013

Posted December 1, 2013, 12:41 p.m. by Matthew Podschweit. [Updated December 13, 2013, 1:55 p.m.]

I arrived at the hospital about 9:45 a.m. today. I slept till 8, I must have needed it. Yesterday's news about MK's MRI really lifted my spirits, but returning to the ICU reminds me that we still have a long road ahead of us. Because of her restlessness, the doctors had to, in essence, paralyze MK in order to get an accurate MRI. In order to keep her breathing, they had to intubate her again. She still has the tube in her throat this morning, and upon waking her, she began flailing around again. She has tossed around so much with the tube in place, that she has caused her throat to swell and they can't remove the tube until the swelling goes down. So now they have to sedate her again, and the cycle continues. I am sitting very quietly beside her bed, wanting to be here for her, but also understanding that stimulating her will cause her to act out more. It's hard to see the light at the end of this tunnel, I trust it's out there somewhere.

I met a woman named Virginia in the waiting room this morning. She came and sat next to me and asked how my loved one was doing. I explained MK's situation, and she shared that her brother-in-law is in ICU awaiting open heart surgery. We visited for a while and we prayed together. It reminded me of when I worked at Heritage and how serving hospital visitation brought me such a sense of purpose and fulfillment. I'm so thankful for all of you that have expressed your love and concern for MK and continue to pray for her.

They are going to keep MK intubated until tomorrow.

At about 1:00 p.m., the neurologist drops by. MK has been still for about ten minutes and this guy busts through the door like a SWAT team, loudly announcing he has arrived and will be examining MK. She immediately wakes and begins flailing around uncontrollably, and I'm having trouble controlling my compulsion to walk him back out of the room by his collar and stuffing his little rubber mallet down his throat. I understand it's going to be necessary to wake her, but how is anyone expected to recover when they can't get uninterrupted sleep?

CHAPTER 15

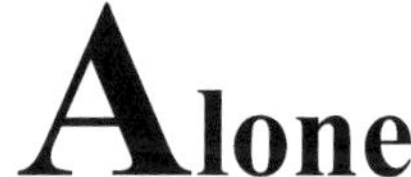

Matt's Blog: Mary Kaye's Odyssey

Monday, December 2, 2013

Posted December 2, 2013, 9:18 p.m. by Matthew Podschweit. [Updated December 13, 2013, 1:55 p.m.]

I returned to work today, but not until I stopped at the hospital. I so badly hoped to walk in to see MK without her breathing tube in, but that was not to be. Dr. Pennington was on the floor and I got to spend some good quality time talking to him. MK is currently being sedated to keep her still. Her throat has been inflamed due to her semi-involuntary reaction to the medicine she is being given. We still haven't determined exactly which medicine might be causing this, but at this point, it's more important to get her extubated and eating some semisolid food. We need to keep her bowels working or her recovery will take much longer.

I basically spent the day catching up to a week's worth of email. Once I had gotten caught up, I headed back to the hospital. MK's nurse today was Uni. She was MK's daytime nurse the first two days she was at St. Francis and quickly became our favorite—just the right balance of drill sergeant and Mother Teresa. MK will need to stay calm and quiet throughout the night so she can be extubated tomorrow. I'll head back tomorrow morning, hoping to see her smile.

Matt's Blog: Mary Kaye's Odyssey

Tuesday, December 3, 2013

Posted December 3, 2013, 11:24 a.m. by Matthew Podschweit. [Updated December 13, 2013, 1:56 p.m.]

I'm at the hospital with MK today. It is 10:00 a.m. and I'm sitting silently next to her bed. She's sleeping peacefully in spite of the nurse's activity around her and the whirring and puffing of the respirator. I'm glad, she really needs to give her throat a rest—it is swollen from the irritation caused by her semi-involuntary movements, and they can't take the breathing tube out until that swelling goes down. She can't start eating until the tube comes out, and if she doesn't start eating, her digestive track will shut down and that will only lengthen her recovery time. I so want to see her beautiful smile.

Home is not home without MK. I've been trying to keep the house clean, hoping it will be more comfortable to be there, but it's cold and quiet and empty. Aubrey is a wonderful companion, and when she's home, everything is better. She has work and school, and needs to see her friends. I miss my true companion and need to stay busy and maintain our household for her sake. I receive a text from my friend Greg just about every day, detailing a Psalm that he prays for MK, and today it is 9:9—the Lord is a shelter for the oppressed, a refuge in times of trouble. He said he prayed this for MK, but it applies to me as well. I will find my shelter in the Lord today, comfort in His faithfulness, belonging in His family, strength in his Spirit.

CHAPTER 16

The Gift to Love Again

Matt's Blog: Mary Kaye's Odyssey

Tuesday, December 3, 2013, continued

Posted December 3, 2013, 11:24 a.m. by Matthew Podschweit. [Updated December 13, 2013, 1:56 p.m.]

At about 10:30 a.m., the nurse came in and shut off all of the medication. She did that to wake MK up because they are taking the breathing tube out. Great news, but I'm still nervous. She has been so peaceful and I'm afraid if they wake her, she'll start writhing around again. I wait for her to start coming around, and she starts to stir. Her eyes open and she's becoming aware of her surroundings. She is uncomfortable, and I'm trying to assure her she's OK and convince her to lie still. About 15 minutes pass (seems more like hours) and finally the doctor, some students and the respiratory therapist come in and remove her breathing tube. Almost instantly, MK is back. Just a few little tics, but she is signing and mouthing words and telling everyone in the room "thank you."

Me

My next memory was December 3, 2013, waking up to Matt singing our song, "I'll Dream of You Again." As he was singing he had to stop because he was so choked up with emotion. So I finished the song, our song. "That's right," he said, "You remember."

I'll Dream of You Again

Song by Harry Connick Jr.

I spent last night dreaming of your eyes

But your hair kept getting in the way

Your lips dropped in to tell me how you'd been

But when I tried to kiss them

My pillow told me I missed them

Your voice dropped by and sang a lullaby

And it was then I knew just what to do

I'd fall asleep and then

I'd dream of you again.

Songwriters: Mirko Von Schlieffen / Peter Heppner / Christopher Von Deylen *I'll Dream of You Again* lyrics © EMI Music Publishing, Warner/Chappell Music, Inc.

When I was in the ICU with Matt and Aubrey, I was trying to ask what day it was. Matt's phone rang and he answered it. While caressing my hand, Aubrey gently said, “Mom, it’s December 3."

Matt shared that Zelda was on the phone and I said, “It’s her birthday!” Matt said, “Whose birthday, honey?” I whispered, “Zelda’s!” He then asked her if it was her birthday and they began to cry. Indeed it was her birthday!

In spite of all my tics and my speech issues Matt was beaming with joy!

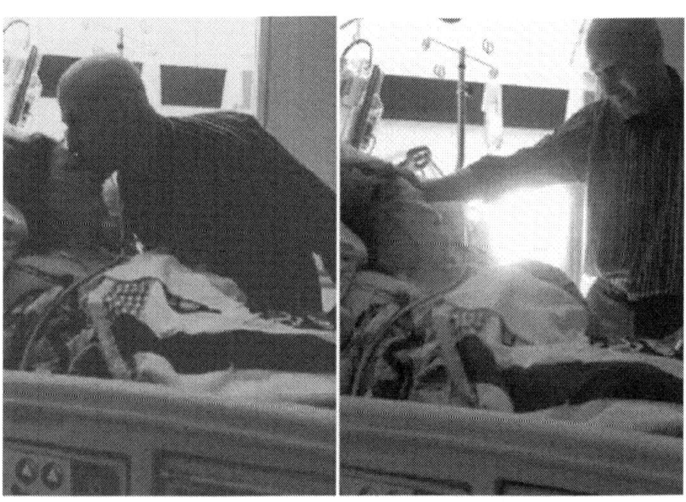

Matt and Mary Kaye

During the time when I was unable to recall anything, spent in the unknown and uncertainty from November 21 thru December 3, my family loved me.

When the outlook was grim, they believed in me!

The times that everything seemed dark and their lives full of despair, they fought for me.

I will hang onto this beautiful time! I will remember when things are difficult, which they will be, how no one gave up on me.

I recall how Jesus held me in his arms and told me I had to go back, that my job was not done. This, I will never forget.

Because of all of this love, I cannot, I will not, give up on myself!

Aubrey

The doctor came in and removed the second breathing tube. Mom's tics were harsh and we weren't sure how much damage had been done. We wouldn't know until she was being forced to breathe on her own.

Tears of joy! The answer was immediate! Mom was awake! She was alive and breathing without assistance and the tics have miraculously stopped!

Dad was overjoyed! I was able to capture on video and witness the beautiful moment of Dad crying over her and singing their song! He became so overwhelmed he couldn't finish. Just then, after the doctors explained that they didn't know how much brain damage had been done due to her uncontrollable muscle movement and the lack of oxygen from CPR, she finished their song! SHE FINISHED THEIR SONG!

Then she was trying to ask what day it was. She was trying to communicate. Once I was able to figure out what she was asking, Dad's phone rang. He answered because it was Zelda, Mom's best friend.

While caressing Mom's hand, I gently said, "Mom, it's December 3." She looked confused.

Dad shared Zelda was on the phone and then Mom quietly said, "It's her birthday."

Dad asked, "Who's birthday, honey?" Mom whispered "Zelda's."

He then asked Zelda if it was her birthday and they began to cry. Indeed it was her birthday!

In spite of all her tics and her speech being slow and monotone, with the fear of brain damage, we were beaming with joy!

Matt's Blog: Mary Kaye's Odyssey

Tuesday, December 3, 2013, continued

Posted December 3, 2013, 11:24 a.m. by Matthew Podschweit. [Updated December 13, 2013, 1:56 p.m.]

It's 11:50 a.m. and MK is taking a breathing treatment to help clear her lungs. She is calmly watching TV and, with the exception of the occasional slight tic, seems to be completely in control of her body. In fact, she seems to have quite a bit of energy. She is signing the alphabet with both hands and carrying on a conversation about it with the respiratory therapist. She is more herself than she's been for twelve days! I'm so thankful that she's off the medication!

CHAPTER 17

Choices

Me

While still in ICU, in and out of consciousness and feeling very confused I began praying. I was trying not to focus on the meditative, hypnotic beeping from the heart monitor. That's when I walked in the garden with Jesus. A picture on the wall came alive—it was breathtaking! The waterfall began streaming, fields of flowers were blooming, and deer were drinking from the pool of water! I saw images of people I once knew but they didn't see me. They were walking along this beautiful trail. I tried to get their attention but I couldn't speak. The waterfall began spilling words, passages from the Scriptures that I have heard many times at funerals.

John 14:3

"And if I go and prepare a place for you, I will come back and take you to be with me that you also may be where I am."

Psalm 23:1–4 A psalm of David

"The Lord is my shepherd, I lack nothing. He makes me lie down in green pastures, he leads me beside quiet waters, he refreshes my soul. He guides me along the right paths for his name's sake. Even though I walk through the darkest valley, I will fear no evil, for you are with me; Your rod and staff, they comfort me."

To me, at that time, I believe God was giving me a choice. I could go and be with Him or I could stay. It was up to me. I laid in bed and cried. I wanted both. He told me in a very gentle way that the decision was mine. It was up to me but He assured me He has never left me nor would He ever leave me. He wanted to use me to share my story, I was given the gift to love again! And that's what I chose, to LOVE! I chose to be the wife to Matt and the mother to our girls. To be the daughter, sister, and friend that God has gifted me to be.

Matt's Blog: Mary Kaye's Odyssey

Wednesday, December 4, 2013

Posted December 4, 2013, 7:28 p.m. by Matthew Podschweit. [Updated December 13, 2013, 1:56 p.m.]

There is not much to report today. MK is doing very well from a medical perspective. Her BP is good, heart rate good, oxygen saturation is excellent. Her tics have completely disappeared and she seems comfortable. She still has some soreness from the bruises around her ribcage and in her belly, but her red blood cell count is not dropping, so it's safe to assume that they are healing. She is down to just IV fluids and her blood pressure medicine, with the occasional oral pain med as needed.

She has been very quiet all day today. I think it's sinking in, the realization of what she's been through. We saw the speech pathologist this afternoon, and she shared that it's common for people in MK's position to get a little depressed—it's perfectly normal, and will get better as we begin speech and memory therapy (tomorrow). I think she also needs some sleep. When I arrived this morning around 9:30 a.m., she told me she hadn't slept at all. I'm going to be kicked out at 6:30 p.m. until 8:00 p.m. for nurse shift change. I'm going to run home and hopefully see Aubrey, and then I 'm going to come back to the hospital for a couple of hours. I can't stand the thought of MK being alone right now. Hopefully she will fall asleep and stay that way until morning.

CHAPTER 18

Out of ICU

Matt's Blog: Mary Kaye's Odyssey

Thursday, December 5, 2013

Posted December 5, 2013, 5:37 p.m. by Matthew Podschweit. [Updated December 13, 2013, 1:56 p.m.]

Today begins at 3:30 a.m. as I wake up with a splitting headache. Not my favorite way to start the day. I had forgotten to take my migraine medicine the night before, better late than never. This set me up for a late start. To make things worse, I got almost all the way to the hospital when I realized I had forgotten my phone. Dang.

I see MK about 9:45 a.m. and I can tell she's already having a better day than yesterday. She's more talkative, and her eyes are a bit brighter. Breakfast is over, but she's working on a cup of Jello, operating the spoon herself. It's almost time for physical therapy, and Jeanette, Rodalyn, and Jimmy come in to facilitate. First, they get MK to her feet with the help of a walker. While she's standing, they have her march in place for a bit. Then, they sit her down in a chair and take her through a few more exercises. After she's finished we sit together and watch a little TV. I flip through the channels looking for something that isn't very emotionally moving, because every time we watch something like Law And Order or Karate Kid, MK starts to cry. I'm looking for a game show or children's programming, maybe Moonshiners or C-SPAN—got to keep that BP down.

The nurse comes in and tells us MK will have a swallow test where she will be x-rayed while she drinks some Barium (yuk!). And after the test, we WON'T be coming back to ICU! Finally, a regular hospital room. Aubrey and I run to Panera while they take MK to her test and then we meet her in room 425. Cozier room, far less equipment and much quieter. This will be much better for sleeping. We anticipate being here only a few more days and then home. That will be an awesome day.

CHAPTER 19

Rebuilding My Life

Matt's Blog: Mary Kaye's Odyssey

Friday, December 6, 2013

Posted December 7, 2013, 9:05 p.m. by Matthew Podschweit. [Updated December 13, 2013, 1:57 p.m.]

This post is late and I apologize. My sister Rhoni came down today to sit with MK while I take care of a few things. I stick around until about 2:00 p.m. and then I'm off. The house is a mess, laundry is piling up and phone calls to the insurance company and the hospital are pending. And I need to go shopping—Aubrey and I have run out of distilled water for the coffee maker, and I know we both have a much better day when it starts off right—with a couple cups of joe.

MK shared a story today—the only memory that she has of this whole trauma. It happened around the time she coded in the ICU at St. Francis. She says she remembers standing in the corner of her room, watching herself being tended to by the hospital staff. She saw Jesus standing in the opposite corner and felt compelled to go to Him, but He told her it was not her time to go. MK said she felt rejected by Jesus. But as I'm sure most people would deduce, I told her Jesus simply still has a purpose for you right here in the world, and has long accepted you as His own.

I've heard some people describe a traumatic event in their lives like this as "testing their faith." I'm not sure I quite understand this analogy. There is no right or wrong answer, no pass/fail evaluation on the conveyor belt. Faith is a choice, yes or no. Regardless of the outcome of your circumstances, you will either choose to trust in the divine purpose of your life, or muddle through on your own.

Me

I was moved to inpatient rehabilitation from ICU at Penrose Hospital in Colorado Springs. It was while I was in rehab that the fear became startling and real. I was an infant in an adult body, truly having to relearn how to...well, everything. It was very difficult not crying in front of my family. They had been and were going through so many changes and were my constant advocates and cheerleaders!

I still had the IV in my neck and a catheter. Each day began with learning how to sit up and to swallow. All of the medicines that I was taking were transported through the IV. The damage to my trachea due to intubation required the therapist to really work with me on rebuilding the muscles used to swallow. My trachea was very sore and a bit swollen so it made that process a little more complicated. But we didn't give up!

CHAPTER 20

Beauty for Ashes

"I know I chose the more difficult path. But there is beauty in ashes and brokenness."
—Mary Kaye

Matt's Blog: Mary Kaye's Odyssey

Saturday, December 7, 2013

Posted December 8, 2013, 7:14 p.m. by Matthew Podschweit. [Updated December 13, 2013, 1:57 p.m.]

What a big day for MK! She is now on the rehab floor and today is her first day of scheduled therapy. Physical therapy from 9:00 a.m. to 10:00 a.m.—after several resistance exercises while sitting on the edge of the bed, MK stood up and walked about 20 ft. out into the hallway. She had planned to make the return trip, but we noticed a pretty significant lightening in her complexion. We sat her down and took her blood pressure—68/40—whoa! Let's get a wheelchair and get her back to bed!

Speech therapy from 10:30 a.m. to 11:30 a.m.—Ken and Paula Gendill, our rock 'n roll friends from Denver, are in town and stop by to say hello. Ken has had his Telecaster with a craftsman here in the Springs for an unprecedented customization and is picking it up today (not sure what a Telecaster is? Google it!). They visit briefly with MK and then the three of us head down to the lobby cafe for a bite to eat while MK works with the speech therapist.

MK eats a light lunch, and then it's time for occupational therapy. The therapist takes MK down the hall for a shower—her first real shower in 16 days. She came back very tired and light-headed, but clean and happy. After all that activity, MK was ready for a rest. I hung out until about 8:00 p.m., and then headed home.

Me

The nurses had explained to me and my family that I was an infant in an adult body. My muscles had gone into atrophy which is why I needed assistance to stand and walk. I also had to relearn how to eat and swallow. I continue to have side effects from this time, all these years later.

I still had the IV in my neck and a catheter. I was not moving on my own and I was still very confused, but everytime my family came to be with me, I smiled! I didn't realize what I had been through and what they had been through, the ups and the downs, the things that haunted them and me. But now, we have hope again! What else can you ask for?

CHAPTER 21

Setbacks and Sleepless Nights

Matt's Blog: Mary Kaye's Odyssey

Sunday, December 8, 2013

Posted December 9, 2013, 8:32 p.m. by Matthew Podschweit. [Updated December 13, 2013, 1:57 p.m.]

7:00 a.m.—I've got to get some work done at home today. I sort and start the laundry and get Aubrey up. She's going to the hospital to sit with MK, and I'm gonna blitz the laundry, kitchen, bills and thank you cards. I'm finding managing the time strangely...well, manageable. Work has been so flexible, Rose, Evan, and Amber have completely taken on the OnDemand coursework help desk, and now that MK is out of ICU, I can ease back in. Our office is very close to the hospital, so I will be able to stop at the hospital before, during lunch, and after pretty conveniently. I need to make sure I'm getting enough sleep, can't get sick.

Today, MK walked about 60 ft. to the nurses' station—exceptional for her second day of therapy, I think. After they got her back in bed, MK noticed swelling in her left leg. It was uncomfortable, painful actually, and we made sure to bring it to her nurse's attention. Her doctor is not in today, so his attention will have to wait. I can tell MK is nervous about it, she's afraid it might be another blood clot. I remind her about the filter in her vena cava and that even if it is a clot, it won't travel to her vital organs, but I know she's still concerned.

We watch the Broncos handle the Titans, and then soon after, I'm off for home—there's still four loads of laundry left and I'm gonna feel better if I can get at least two of them done before bed. MK is very sleepy—I kiss her on the forehead, tell her I love her, and leave feeling confident that tomorrow will bring a little more progress and a little closer to MK coming home.

Matt's Blog: Mary Kaye's Odyssey

Monday, December 9, 2013

Posted December 9, 2013, 8:55 p.m. by Matthew Podschweit. [Updated December 13, 2013, 1:58 p.m.]

Time to try out my work/hospital routine. I'm gonna try to get to the hospital by 7:00 a.m. OK, that would have gone better if I'd have gotten out of bed before 6:20 a.m. At least I remembered the outgoing mail, to take the garbage to the curb, and I even packed my lunch. I get there before 8:00 a.m. and get to meet Dr. House. Yup, for real. He lets us know that he has scheduled an ultrasound to see what's going on with MK's leg. I decide to stay until they do the test. A quick email to my coworkers, and then down to radiology. The test takes a while, and I answer a few emails while Sara the technician conducts the scan. Pretty cool gear, I think in another life I might enjoy learning how to use it. We head back up to MK's room, and the results won't be back until after lunch. I head back to work, planning to join MK for lunch.

I arrive back at the hospital at 12:45 p.m., but no results yet. MK has just gotten her tray, so I unpack my lunch and we eat together. After we finish, KJ the speech therapist comes in and takes MK through her list of words that end with a hard "k" sound—bake, cook, look, etc. She is supposed to hit the ending consonant really hard, as if she was a cat hacking up a hairball. Sounds like fun, and so I join in. But enough frivolity, this is serious therapy. I head back to work.

I get back to the hospital about 6:00 p.m. MK tells me the ultrasound shows two blood clots in MK's left leg. This is not a crisis, but is making MK quite uncomfortable (both physically and emotionally—can't blame her). I ask her nurse to explain the test results, and she says she doesn't have them. OK, now I'm confused. Guess I'll wait to see Dr.

House in the morning. After dinner, MK is sleeping soundly—the Bears play the Cowboys on Monday Night Football tonight, think I'll let MK sleep and try to catch the game. And I'd better make sure to get to the hospital by 7:00 a.m. tomorrow.

Me

December 10

Matt would come in at least twice a day, assisting when he could. He was always smiling and so happy. Even when I felt I had a setback he believed in me. My left leg was swollen and still felt warm. The thought of having blood clots again made sleeping impossible. This is when the nightmares started.

I was so very tired all of the time. All alone in my room, I would focus on putting names and faces together. I remember trying to rest, to embrace the love I had from my family, and convince myself I was alive. This was real. I was startled awake at 3:30 a.m. unable to breathe and unable to move.

Then the nightmares got much worse and very graphic. I experienced the feeling of being tied down, unable to move, unable to breathe as horrific beasts manipulated me and my body. Scared, no, horrified, yes. I was fearful of falling asleep.

I still struggled with the realization that something happened. I would ask about it often as best as I could. Communication was still incredibly difficult. I would try to form words but my speech was very soft and monotone.

December 11

I struggled with nightmares but was not able to share what I was experiencing, unsure myself how to verbalize it. It was always a feeling of being tied down and unable to breathe. I would wake up periodically in tears, but unable to say anything. The staff would come in and check on me often because while I was sleeping my heart would begin to race and my tics became worse. It was all of these symptoms that led the staff to believe it was hallucinations, which is common from an extended period in ICU. Sometimes these dreams and hallucinations caused anxiety, confusion, or disorientation. I found it difficult to distinguish between dreams, nightmares, and hallucinations particularly when I first came round. These dreams could be unpleasant, strange, and frightening.

I was so fearful of falling asleep. One of the nurse's aides would come into my room every night at 3:30 a.m. She would hold my hand and pray over me, and with me. I believed her name was Mary. She would talk very slowly and had an incredibly gentle spirit. It wasn't until after she left me that I was able to get some much-needed rest.

CHAPTER 22

Juggling

Matt's Blog: Mary Kaye's Odyssey

Thursday, December 12, 2013

Posted December 12, 2013, 10:12 p.m. by Matthew Podschweit.

I am very sorry for leaving you hanging—this hospital/work schedule has left me little time to think let alone write. The doctors in the ICU used to tell us "no news is good news" and I'm glad to say it applies.

MK's physical and occupational therapy is hard work. She has been out of bed, standing, a little walking, lots of exercises and back and forth to the shower room a couple of times. She gets 3-4 hours of therapy every day, and to say she is pooped by dinner time is an understatement. MK seems to be experiencing less discomfort associated with the clots in her left leg, which would seem to indicate they are beginning to be absorbed. She is working SO HARD. All good.

The team has given MK a target discharge date of December 19, which may be a little ambitious, but certainly gives us great hope that she'll be home before Christmas.

CHAPTER 23

Visitors in the Night

Me

December 13

Pastor Rick from the hospital would often come and visit with me. When I was able to speak about my conversation with Jesus and how I felt so rejected because He sent me back, he listened and then would smile. I remember asking him one day why he smiled when I shared my heartache and he patiently said, "I come and visit with you every day. And every day you share the same experience. You cry when you say *rejected*. And every day I listen and tell you that Jesus knows your heart and how you feel rejected because HE too was rejected. And every day we pray that you will understand HIS love for you and how HIS plan is greater in your life than you can see."

"Every day?" I ask. "We've had this conversation before?" "Every day," he said. Then he asks if I can tell him what happened. (I sigh.) Trying to stay positive with the outlook was becoming exhausting. I never wanted my family to see how emotionally draining all of this was, and I understood how hard this had been for everyone.

The inpatient rehab staff would often comment on my pleasant disposition. Most said it was good but Dr. House wanted more of a fight. I just didn't know if I could fight—I just wanted to coast for a while.

December 14

My day starts early with 7:30 physical therapy. Today it was learning how to sit down in bed and get back up on my own. Something so simple. Well, it used to be anyway.

I began to rely on my nightly visits with Mary. She always knew what to ask and was so incredibly patient with me. Sometimes I was not able to articulate how I was feeling, but this did not stop her from loving me and helping me through the night.

After all of my therapy sessions Matt came to spend the afternoon with me. I could tell all of this was taking a toll on him. He looked weary.

When he asked how I was sleeping I looked down at my hands on my lap. I didn't want to bother him with my fears. He then came over and knelt beside me, lifted my chin and wiped the tears from my eyes. "Honey," he said gently, "what's wrong?"

I took a deep breath and shared with him about my nightmares and how I was scared to fall asleep. Up until now, I had never told him about how Mary, the nurse's aide would come in and pray with me. I never mentioned how 3:30 a.m. was the peak of terrors. I would wake up wanting to scream but I had no voice. There was only the ticking of the clock on the wall.

Matt said, "I'll help sweetie, please don't cry."

Aubrey

Dad shared about Mom's nightmares. I asked him if it would be okay for me to visit after work. He wasn't sure because they close the doors at 9 p.m. and I worked late, but he said maybe they would let me in.

I was going to be the compassionate daughter that Mom always thinks I am. I was going to help her through this difficult time.

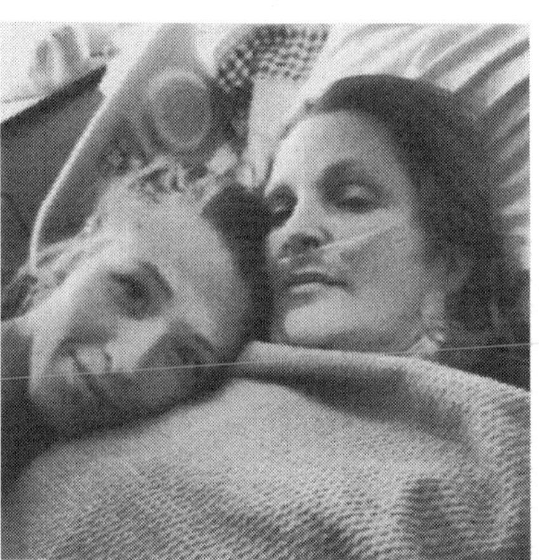

Aubrey and Mary Kaye

Me

December 15

That morning I awoke to Aubrey nestled next to me at 2 a.m. She came to the hospital after work. I was so glad she was there. She was with me. It helped with the realization that I was alive. I had closed my eyes, holding this precious girl, this beautiful daughter God has blessed us with.

I still awoke at 3:30 a.m., this time to Mary standing over us smiling. She tucked Aubrey in and said a quiet prayer. I closed my eyes.

Then I woke up at 6:30 a.m. to get ready for a new day. Aubrey was not there but left a beautiful note for me, her way of letting me know she loves me.

"*There is only one true happiness in this life. That is to love and be loved. Thank you for still being here.*" She signed it, "*Love, your favorite daughter, Aubrey.*"

CHAPTER 24

Fatigue and Disappointment

Me

December 16

Inpatient rehab was incredibly difficult. All of it.

Speech Therapy

I was probably the easiest patient simply because I was too weak to fight. I dreaded therapy. Every day I had speech, occupational, and physical therapy.

The staff would write on the blackboard in my room the day's agenda and in turn I would have to read out loud what it said. The comprehension of letters and sound was very difficult. I could read what was on the board but to articulate what was written was impossible, seemed impossible. I had lost my tone and diction. I was only able to speak in whispers. Simple cards for preschoolers, naming colors, numbers, and simple words like dog and cat stumped me. I grew very tired of this process. I was able to recognize family and friends but to say their names was very confusing. The speech therapist would hold up the card for dog. I was asked to name each letter. *"Deee Deee Deee Deee."* Sigh. Deep breath. *"OooooOoooOoooOooo."* Sigh. Breathe. *"Gaaaagaaaagaaa."* The speech therapist would correct me and say not the sound but the letter. *"Gaaagaaagaaagaaa."*

Tears streamed down my face because I was mentally exhausted and lost common knowledge of simple words and understanding how to verbally communicate what I was reading.

Occupational Therapy

I had to relearn to take care of personal hygiene. I had to relearn how to shower, brush my teeth, and comb my hair. Eventually, I was "forced" in the kitchen and had to cook macaroni and cheese. Which of course everyone in my family had a good laugh at since I hated the kitchen before I got sick.

Everything was exhausting. Showering was most difficult. My blood pressure would suddenly drop which in turn startled the staff. I recall one shower I was not able to finish because I blacked out. Thank goodness a nurse was always with me and so was my occupational therapist so they whisked me in a wheelchair back to my room and tucked me into bed until my heart rate stabilized.

During occupational therapy I always thought that was the worst part of my day. I grew very tired of this process. I would try to remember how to care for myself, brush my teeth and hair. As excited as my family was, I was crying inside. Fear was real.

Physical Therapy

Or torture therapy was the worst of them all, having to relearn how to walk and use my arms, hands, and feet all over again. My brain did not want to connect to my extremities. I relied on my wheelchair and walker for quite awhile. The therapists were relentless. Although I did not want to do the demanding tasks of learning how to sit up and then sit back down, they did not give up.

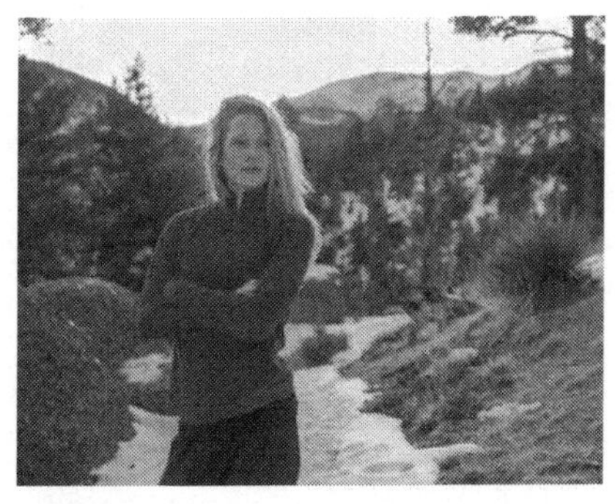

Emily

Emily came home for her break and came directly to rehab. I had both of my cheerleaders there with me. I didn't know how we would handle the much-needed rehab but I knew we could do it all together!

The game plan was to get me home December 17, tomorrow! But the doctors would not release me. The excitement and the disappointment was all over the place. I needed a game plan so Greg, the head of PT, wrote it on the blackboard for me… once again I had to read. I had to put letters together to form words. I had to comprehend what was going on. I was still on and off of oxygen. They were able to remove the catheter and finally remove the IV from my neck. But part of the problems I was facing was learning how to void and use the bathroom. The nurses had explained to me and my family that I was an infant in an adult body. I had to relearn how to eat and swallow. I had lots of work to do.

Matt's Blog: Mary Kaye's Odyssey

Tuesday, December 17, 2013

Posted December 17, 2013, 10:07 p.m. by Matthew Podschweit.

Today we heard from Dr. House that they are pushing back MK's discharge date to December 31. Christmas will be celebrated in room 808 at Penrose Main. Poor MK, wants nothing more than to be home, the sooner the better. She was quite upset when Dr. House delivered the news. Thankfully Aubrey, Emily, and Colby (Emily's boyfriend) were there at the time and softened the blow (a talent I'd like to think they have inherited from their father).

When I visit MK after work, I reassure her that this is not her fault, and that this is not an injustice being masochistically exercised by the hospital staff. It is what it is. And this is not something that has happened to just MK, but something that has happened to us. We will get through this together, no matter how long it takes.

The primary reason for the extended stay in room 808 is managing MK's blood pressure. In an effort to get a better handle on it, Dr. House is going to discontinue her blood pressure medicine, at least for a time. Her BP has been regularly dropping like a stone when she stands to walk. She does well for a minute, and then she becomes very dizzy and must sit. Behold, our next hurdle.

CHAPTER 25

There's Something About Rhoni

Me

December 18

After the news of extending my stay, I felt incredibly discouraged. I wasn't wanting to show the disappointment to my family, although Matt knew just by seeing me how heavy my heart was.

Rhoni came to visit for the day. I love seeing her. She is always so very animated and can make a bad day worse...I mean better, she can make a bad day better!

We were visiting after all of my therapy appointments when Dr. G (that's what everyone called him. I really don't know his actual name) came into my room. He had asked Rhoni to step outside so we could talk. Rhoni got up and said, "I'll be back in a few minutes, pretty lady."

I looked very confused and said, "What did you just say?"

Poor Rhoni looked rather dejected and said loudly, like I couldn't hear her the first time, "I'll be back." She looked at Dr. G very concerned that something was happening! I smile at her and laughingly say, "No, not that part, the pretty lady part!" She belly laughed; we all did. She walked out of the room lighthearted, saying, "She's back!"

CHAPTER 26

Mother's Love

Me

December 19

After another brain scan, the neurologist explained that my brain was permanently damaged and some things I used to do without thought will be difficult. I have lots of work to do. She explained it's not a surprise but she believes we, as a family, can and will find a way to embrace this new speed of life. Honestly, I know she was trying to be optimistic, but darn...not what I wanted to hear.

Judy

It was my scheduled turn to come and sit with Mary because Matt had to go back to work. I didn't mind because I had the chance to watch our Mary work so hard, and I found a new appreciation for my darling girl! So I would bring my knitting and would sit and knit while Mary did all of her therapy. When she came back to the room I would always read her a story. Mary would make comments about how her mom would crochet, and how she cherished everything that she received from her. Talking about Mary's mom, Karen, made Mary look very sad. She needed her mom. I asked her if she would like me to call Mom, and she gently nodded her head yes. Karen answered on the first ring and I talked to her briefly before I gave the phone to Mary, then I left the room so that they could have some privacy.

Karen

I was so happy to hear from Judy, but more importantly to hear my sweet Mary's voice. She was very soft spoken and I was doing most of the talking. Maybe it was nervous talking, I am not sure. Either way, I was so happy to be on the phone with her. It had been so long since I had talked with her. Mary was able to ask me to sing a song to her and I knew just what song to sing, "*You are my sunshine,*" I began. It was exactly what both of us needed.

CHAPTER 27

The Significance of 3:30 a.m.

Me

December 20

I looked forward to my daily visits from Pastor Rick. He brought so much comfort and didn't mind me repeating myself over and over and over again. He became a friend. He was so close that he knew at 3:00 I was spent. I was in bed and watching The Ellen DeGeneres Show sometimes and he would come into the room and watch with me. Then he would ask me something about the show, trying to get me to talk and repeat something I just watched. Personally, I think Ellen should be on everyone's agenda. Always loving, smiling, and laughing! When she danced I would move my feet to the music, and anyone who came to visit from 3-4 had to watch with me! I tried to memorize her jokes and repeat them—I certainly did not do a good job with that, but nonetheless, I would try! Trying to memorize and repeat it with my lack of speech certainly did create lots of laughter!

I told him about my nightmares and that they usually began around 3:30 a.m. and how Mary would come in and pray. He looked astonished and pleased that a staff member cared so deeply to take the time and find a way to ease the fears that the nightmares brought.

I always shared the same stories about the nightmares and my time with Jesus. It was Pastor Rick who put the time frame together for me and helped me understand why 3:30 a.m. was so significant. He told me that his thought was that it was at that time when Jesus was holding me and I wasn't afraid of dying. Also, 3:30 a.m. was the time I had last coded. It was at 3:30 a.m. that Jesus sent me back and I felt rejected. It was at that time I was comforted by Jesus and scared to go back. But now, I was scared of dying, of not being the wife to Matt, and the mother to our two beautiful girls. It's love that makes this journey messy, beautiful, and joyful.

There was a birthday in my family today and I was able to wish my beautiful niece, Amanda, a happy birthday! Amanda is David and Carla's youngest daughter. Both Megan and Amanda were amazing during this time. The love they both have for their parents is truly a gift. Thanks for sharing the love with me and my family. David and Carla continued to keep in close communication with Matt and keep their daughters informed of my progress.

December 21

I was able to participate in the Great Room Activities just down the hall from my room. I was still using a wheelchair but I was happy to have something else to do. We were having an art therapy session and we were instructed to make a Christmas card. Everyone was making their cards and then I remembered it was my incredibly talented and very loving niece's birthday, Alex (Rhoni and David's daughter)! So instead of following instructions, I did my own thing! The art instructor was not very happy with me for not following instructions, but I didn't care! Surprise, surprise, a bit of the old Mary Kaye is coming back! Watch out world here I come! I couldn't wait to give Alex the card that I had made for her! The family was planning a Christmas party in rehab and I would see her then and give her the card!

CHAPTER 28

Dance for Joy

Me

December 24

It was Christmas Eve. I was laying in bed in silence, feeling alone, unsure, confused, and scared of what the future holds. Sometimes, the quiet was beautiful and other times it was scary. This was scary silence. I was still afraid to sleep because of the haunting nightmares and unable to tell anyone except Pastor Rick, or simply scared to. I was thinking something was wrong with me. My family had all come up earlier that morning between rehabilitation sessions, and I knew I would be alone for the rest of the day. I prayed for God to help me out of this sadness, and for some rest. I didn't want my family or friends to see me feeling sad. I was afraid. That was the day it all came to me: this was going to be a long and difficult road. I would never be able to live my life like I knew it before the scattered memory of my past. How could my husband love me? How could I be a mother and someday a grandma? What life would I live, how could Matt ever be happy with a disabled wife? Yup, I was feeling sorry for myself.

I heard singing in the hallway and smiled at all the times music brought great comfort. There was a knock on my door and a heavenly choir came in! Pastor Rick had asked for his church choir to do hospital visits and put me on the list. They prayed with me and sang "Silent Night"! It was so beautiful, so very peaceful. Peace, the beauty of answered prayers. Something so simple, so personal, so lovely.

Silent night, holy night!

All is calm, all is bright.

Round yon Virgin, Mother and Child.

Holy infant so tender and mild,

Sleep in heavenly peace,

Sleep in heavenly peace.

Silent night, holy night!

Shepherds quake at the sight.

Glories stream from heaven afar

Heavenly hosts sing Alleluia,

Christ the Savior is born!

Christ the Savior is born.

Silent night, holy night!
Son of God love's pure light.
Radiant beams from Thy holy face
With the dawn of redeeming grace,
Jesus Lord, at Thy birth
Jesus Lord, at Thy birth.

Silent night, holy night,
All is calm, all is bright
Round yon virgin mother and child.
Holy infant so tender and mild,
Sleep in heavenly peace.
Sleep in heavenly peace.

After their visit and precious songs, I finally got a good night's sleep!

December 25

I remember waking up at 3:30 a.m. and seeing Mary praying a prayer of gratitude over me. I fell asleep once again, I think this time with a smile on my face.

Christmas Day I still had rehab scheduled. My family was decorating the conference room and preparing a party. We all dressed in Hello Kitty PJs in memory of Phil! He passed away in September (Phil came to visit me when I coded. I will always be very grateful for that time. His message was to *"Be sure to tell Judy that I love her"*). Phil had an ongoing joke about Hello Kitty, so I was glad that everyone honored his memory with wearing Hello Kitty PJs on Christmas morning. I am sure he loved it as well!

When I was walking the hallway using a walker, I went the farthest that day without stopping. A new day of hope, a new day of challenges, and a new day of conquering obstacles. God had blessed me with a competitive spirit and I had to find that, for my family. I had to live, to love, and to laugh. I was not going to settle. This was not going to be my normal.

When my niece Alex saw me walking with a walker she began dancing in the hallway full of excitement! I stopped. My physical therapist said, "Are you okay?" I said joyfully, "I am alive!"

CHAPTER 29

40 Days in the Wilderness

December 26

With a new energy and game plan, I became determined to try no matter what obstacle they placed in front of me. I would fight the fears and work hard. Building endurance was very difficult. We were still trying to manage my heart rate. When I felt dizzy I would just stop until I felt I could get up and try again. The mechanics of walking were difficult. But the PT team knew I wanted to be pushed. They decided to try stairs. I cried. I wasn't ready. Greg wasn't buying the tears. He said, "We are doing this today. If it takes all day and all night we will do this!" He was so serious I knew I had to try. With my right hand I held on to the railing. One student was in front and one in the back. Greg was on my left side. It was only eleven steps. Only eleven down and up. Only eleven steps that took a full hour and exhaustion trying to pick up my feet and climb. My brain had to continue to reset. What I mean by that is it would remember to take a step up or down and then reboot. Leaving me guessing. We did it. I don't believe anyone was happy with the outcome. He said we would do it again tomorrow. (*Sigh.*)

Greg had called Matt and shared with him the game plan and asked if he would bring tennis shoes, and if Aubrey and Emily could join him and his team tomorrow.

December 27

Sure enough, everyone was there! Greg shared that we were going to walk outside and that Matt had brought tennis shoes for me. I cried and said, "I can't, I'm not ready." Then like a gentle slap, I was reminded of Philippians 4:13, "I can do all things through Christ who gives me strength" (Berean Study Bible).

Walking outside, breathing the cool, crisp, December air, was overwhelming. I just wanted to cry. I felt tortured. I just didn't know how to articulate my discomfort. I would go about four steps and then stop because I simply forgot how to pick up my feet. Someone would coach me and tell me to pick up my right foot and then show me which is my right foot, and I would then pick up my right foot and then my left and forget again. As excited as my family was to see me vertical and outside, I was dying on the inside. Doubt was overwhelming, swallowing me. The only thing that got me through was knowing Jesus' words to me, "*Your job is not done.*" Knowing that I could not be useful in this state gave me more of a reason to work hard. My family never stopped believing in me and I had to be prepared for the hard work.

December 28

I had begun refusing to use the wheelchair and used only the walker. The staff would have someone go behind me pushing the chair as I was trying to stay with the walker. As I was fighting for this right with the little voice I had, I was sent to my room. Yes, I was being scolded. I then refused to go back to bed so I sat up in the recliner. Who knew I had a stubborn side?

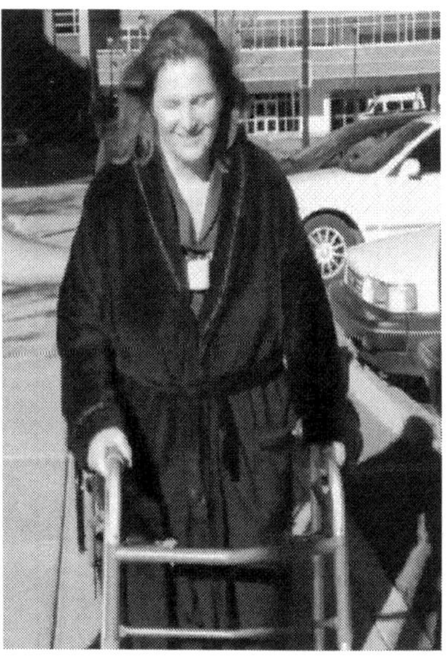

Zelda knew. And guess who came to see me? Zelda and her family all piled into my room! Zelda cheered on my stubborness! She understood that to take some control over my life was a good thing. It was so great to see her! She laughed that I could remember her birthday, December 3, but had no memory of what I had for breakfast!

That afternoon Pastor Rick and Matt were visiting. Dr. House came into my room and shared that I was going home on December 31 as scheduled. Matt was beaming! "I knew you could do it, love!"

Jokingly, Dr. House shared, "It will be forty days on the thirty-first since you came into the hospital and if you stay any longer they will have to start charging you rent!" Pastor Rick and Matt laughed! Then Dr. House and Pastor Rick left the room. Now it was just Matt and me.

Matt reached over to my hand and gently said, "Honey, what's wrong?"

I said in a hoarse whisper, "Forty days? I feel like I have been lost. Forty days of my life that I struggle with remembering. Forty days of fighting to be back to you, and I'm broken, I'll never be the same person. It's been forty days and I still struggle with understanding what happened." Now tears were streaming.

Matt gently kissed my hand and said, "I feel like you were lost, we almost lost you forever. It's like you were trying to find your way home in the wilderness, but we never gave up, we were searching for you, hoping you could hear us. No one stopped believing, no one stopped loving, and no one stopped praying that you would find your way back to us."

"Honey," Matt said, "I've kept a blog to let everyone know what we needed. So many amazing people have been on this journey with you, with us. I thought I was writing it for them but I think I was writing it for you too."

"Forty days?" I whisper.

"Forty days in the wilderness, lost, and you came back!" Matt said with a huge smile! "We are going home!"

Matt then reminded me of the biblical significance of forty days. I was amazed. He shared that the number forty in the Bible has to do with times of testing or hardship. He said we would have to look all of them up in the Old and New Testament when I was ready.

I am so humbled that God has been with me, with us, this whole time. He never left us, and we have never stopped looking to Him.

CHAPTER 30

Love Wins

December 29

As I was preparing for my final days in rehab, I wanted to be sure and thank everyone for their attention and help. When I asked if I could thank Mary personally for her care during the night shift, they looked puzzled and explained that they didn't have a Mary working that shift. I just smiled and closed my eyes and thanked God for Mary, my angel.

Emily and Aubrey worked on helping me finding a new normal. During Christmas break, I think Emily spent most of her time with me learning how to help me.

As part of my memory therapy, Emily would have me remember a simple joke or something from watching Ellen and repeat it back to her. (I am pretty sure this is how the telephone game was invented!) She did this at a time in her life when she should have been taking chances, making mistakes, and getting messy, but there she stood beside me!

I am forever grateful for the encouragement, love, and unyielding support that both Aubrey and Emily have given to me.

Matt's Blog: Mary Kaye's Odyssey

Sunday, December 29, 2013

Posted December 29, 2013, 10:40 p.m. by Matthew Podschweit. [Updated December 29, 2013, 10:40 p.m.]

It has been a long time since my last post, but please don't think that not much has been happening. MK has been working so hard at physical and occupational therapy, and it's all about to pay off. Her discharge date of December 31 is still in force, and if you ask her, MK will tell you it can't come soon enough! This is not a reflection of the care she is receiving at Penrose Main Hospital—in fact, I think MK would agree that we will miss the wonderful people that have been instrumental in getting her prepared to come home.

Each day of therapy brings more and more progress. MK spent so much time in ICU, much of it on a ventilator. Many of her muscles, including her diaphragm, have atrophied to a certain extent. Dr. Guerrero, one of MK's doctors for rehab, reminded us that she may have spent as much as twelve minutes without a constant supply of oxygen to her brain. While her MRI did not show any permanent brain damage, that kind of injury will take time and effort to heal. Right now, MK is able to perform basic, everyday tasks and is walking very well with the assistance of a walker or cane. Her speech has been most noticeably affected. Physically, her time with the breathing tube has damaged her vocal cords and the muscles in her throat. Her voice is very quiet and breathy, and she needs to put much effort into projecting. She also becomes frustrated, as vocalizing what is in her mind is sometimes very difficult. We have been assured that none of this is necessarily permanent and that time and patience along with hard work in therapy will restore MK's abilities.

Throughout this chapter, our family has been the recipient of extraordinary grace and generosity. Expressions of love in the form of prayers and well-wishes, calls and visits, offers of service and help, and providence of food and money have overwhelmed and humbled us beyond my ability to express. Our deepest, heartfelt thanks go out to the many family and friends who have come alongside and shouldered this effort with us.

I resist the temptation to refer to our current situation as a "burden" or a "tragedy" because it is not as long as we think otherwise. Every day brings new opportunities to nurture relationships, to encourage and uplift each other and foster an environment of love and cooperation. To allow ourselves to become mired in woe and self-pity would undermine what I consider to be the most worthwhile purpose of our lives—to sacrificially infuse love as an antidote into a culture that is poisoning itself with greed, selfishness, and hate. It starts at home, and I choose to love MK more tomorrow than I did today, and (thankfully) she chooses to do the same to me. I'd be hard pressed to find anything to complain about.

It occurred to me that as MK returns home, it might be a good idea to ask her to take over this blog. I'll let you know her answer in a future post—please stay tuned.

Love wins!

(Back cover)

Broken Hallelujah is an engaging and true account of the journey of Mary Kaye (MK) and Matt Podschweit and will touch you in the depths of your heart!

Mary Kaye died three times, and was left with an Anoxic Brain Injury (ABI) from a Pulmonary Embolism. You will be engulfed in the struggles and emotional ups and downs that her family and friends endured; the pressure in the midst of making so many quick decisions and responses that were necessary to save her life; and how her fight from traumatic events in her past gave her the strength to fight for her life when faced with so many challenges.

Some of the things they share will leave you weeping!

Some events are very raw and brutally honest!

Some will make you laugh out loud!

Some will restore your hope in people, in love, and in family!

You are invited to be a part of this riveting story and maybe find a bit of yourself in it. May the truth of it bring freedom from fear and past pain and light your path to hope.

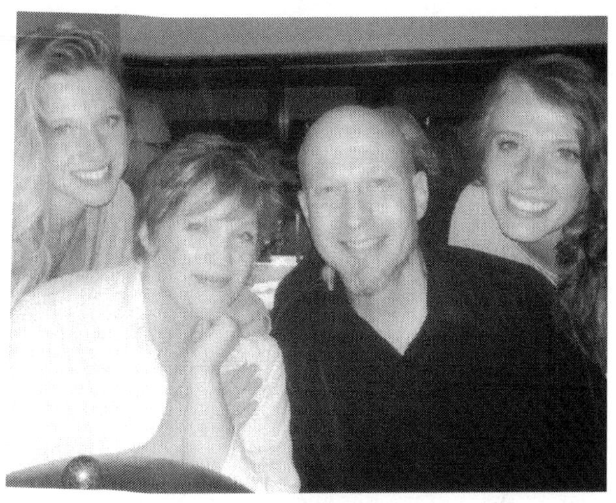

Podschweit Family
Left to Right
Emily, MK, Matt, and Aubrey

Book Cover design by
Tammy Bennett www.tammybennett.myportfolio.com
Original Artwork by
MK Podschweit
Titled "Lean on Me"
As a reflection of her relationship with her husband, Matt

Made in the USA
Monee, IL
11 March 2020

23047044R00129